Praise for *The Day I Die*

"Anita Hannig bravely takes on a topic that many won't touch with a ten-foot pole. Medical aid in dying might be controversial, but it is increasingly accepted worldwide and a topic we can no longer ignore."

—Jessica Zitter, MD, MPH, author of *Extreme Measures: Finding a Better Path to the End of Life* and founder of Do No Harm Media

"Of all events in a lifetime, death is the most solitary, and yet most people have no control over it. In *The Day I Die*, Anita Hannig investigates assisted dying. Her portrayal of people who want to have a choice at the end of their lives is calm, balanced, and devastating."

—Sallie Tisdale, author of *Advice for Future Corpses*

"By sharing the accounts of terminally ill individuals from all walks of life, Anita Hannig provides an honest look at the vital importance of medical aid in dying. From the perspective of patients, physicians, and family members alike, the one immutable truth that resonates is that the desire to experience a good death is simply the extension of having lived a good life. In *The Day I Die*, Hannig helps us recognize that, in our final chapter of life, we are likely to find our collective humanity as much as our inevitable mortality."

—Dan Diaz, Brittany Maynard's husband and advocate for end-of-life options

"*The Day I Die* is the book we need on the next major social issue of our time—a revelation."

—Peter Richardson, director of *How to Die in Oregon*

"Anita Hannig presents both the history of medical aid in dying in the United States and the current reality facing individuals who wish to end their suffering in compassionate and vivid prose. With all her training and hands-on experience, she brings us details of real people trying to end their lives when they realize that nothing but misery lies ahead. Copies of this book should be in every doctor's office in the country to educate patients and doctors themselves!"

—Diane Rehm, interviewer and narrator of the
PBS documentary *When My Time Comes*

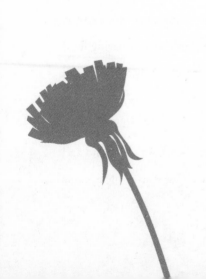
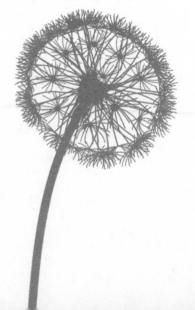

The
Day
I Die

THE UNTOLD STORY OF
ASSISTED DYING IN AMERICA

ANITA HANNIG

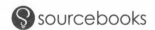

Published by Sourcebooks
P.O. Box 4410, Naperville, Illinois 60567-4410
(630) 961-3900
sourcebooks.com

Library of Congress Cataloging-in-Publication Data

Names: Hannig, Anita, author.
Title: The day I die : the untold story of assisted dying in America /
    Anita Hannig.
Description: Naperville, Illinois : Sourcebooks, [2022] | Includes
    bibliographical references.
Identifiers: LCCN 2021052668 (print) | LCCN 2021052669 (ebook) |
Subjects: LCSH: Assisted suicide. | Assisted suicide--United States.
Classification: LCC R726 .H36 2022 (print) | LCC R726 (ebook) | DDC
    364.152/3--dc23/eng/20211227
LC record available at https://lccn.loc.gov/2021052668
LC ebook record available at https://lccn.loc.gov/2021052669

Printed and bound in the United States of America.
VP 10 9 8 7 6 5 4 3 2 1

To Derianna,
trailblazer extraordinaire

Disease lays me down on worn bedsheets.
Then, as if my hope were enough, she raises me.

From her hand I eat pears with salt.
I follow her into a maze of wordless candor.

She leads me away
from the promise of ripening grass

to fields withered with frost, where swollen soil
is punctured by voles' blind certainties.

She anoints my head with cold rain.
No hour is an hour when she is finished.

Again and again I sun myself,
counting the days of my life.

SAM SESKIN, TO HAVE BEEN SNOWED ON

Table of Contents

Author's Note

This is a work of narrative nonfiction. All events took place exactly as they are described. There are no composite characters or fictional elements. However, with a few exceptions, the names of patients and their loved ones have been changed to protect their privacy. I omitted last names for the same reason. In some cases, the names of physicians were altered, as were some locations to prevent easy identification of individual patients. All errors are mine.

Nothin' about the Blues

The morning of Ken's death, I stood in front of my closet, trying to figure out what to wear. I knew Ken didn't want his death to be a somber affair. He was ready, giddy even. The drab librarian dress was definitely out. Jeans, on the other hand, seemed a little too casual. I wanted to look nice and give Ken's death the gravity it deserved, while also honoring his wish to celebrate. As I thumbed through my hangers, I couldn't help but feel the dissonance of choosing an outfit for someone's final hours. Three years into my research on assisted dying, I still found myself in situations like this with no formal playbook. But if I didn't decide promptly, I was going to be late. Finally, I opted for a pair of striped summer slacks, a sleeveless, navy-blue satin blouse, and leather sandals. Then I grabbed my notebook and ran out the door.

Thirty blocks to the east, at the foot of one of Portland's iconic city parks, Ken was also getting ready. Though he had spent much of his life flaunting propriety, he had decided to dress up for his death. In the quiet light of the morning, he trimmed his white Vandyke beard, slipped into a clean pair of khakis, buttoned his olive-colored dress shirt, and threw on a charcoal vest. He dug out his red bandanna and tied it in a neat triangle knot around his neck. Then he traded his tired plaid house slippers for a pair of elegant, pointy leather brogues.

Ken's breakfast that day was simple: a single hard-boiled egg and a cup of black coffee laced with Fireball whiskey. Not that it was his habit to drink alcohol with breakfast—it didn't mix well with his heart medications—but today Ken felt festive. He had waited for this day for months.

At 10:30 a.m., I met Ken's prescribing physician, Neil Martin, in the foyer of Ken's retirement facility. Save for his medical bag, which could have passed for a plump briefcase, you wouldn't have guessed Martin was a doctor—he wore a cornflower-blue dress shirt, black Levi's, and hiking sneakers. Martin had begun working with terminally ill patients interested in using Oregon's Death with Dignity law in 2009. After his retirement from family medicine in 2015, he had kept his license so he could continue to volunteer as a physician.

Martin and I signed the facility's guest log and made our way to Ken's apartment in the far corner of the building. At the entrance to the dining hall, next to a roster of activity charts announcing bingo night and water aerobics, a cluster of walkers sat parked, waiting for their owners to return. We swung a left down a wide hallway lined with rustic watercolor paintings all depicting stone bridges reaching across gurgling creeks. The pictures conjured a pleasant but generic nostalgia. Ken couldn't stand them.

When we entered his apartment, everyone else was already there: Ken and his two sons, Tony and Zack; Ken's granddaughter, who had flown in from California; and Sophie, his beloved caregiver. Standing and chatting among the family was Derianna Mooney, a volunteer for End of Life Choices Oregon—a nonprofit that accompanies patients and families on their path to an assisted death. Derianna was here to ensure that everything went smoothly and that Ken felt supported in his wish to die.

The apartment looked exactly like it had the last time I was there: stuffed with furniture, unwieldy plants, Ken's hand-drawn paintings, and stacks of loose paper. Two golden helium balloons—spelling 90—still clung, bloated, to the ceiling like giant bubbles trapped under a bottle cap. Ken had turned ninety exactly a week ago.

In the years leading up to his ninetieth birthday, Ken had gone from living in a house in Southern California he shared with his wife, Clara, to living with her in a sheltered but intolerably dull retirement complex in Portland to living alone after he had to admit her to a memory care facility. Worried about their dad's declining health and their mom's progressive dementia, their sons had persuaded Ken and Clara to sell their house near San Bernardino and move up to Portland to be closer to them. For the first six years after their move, Ken had taken care of Clara himself in their shared one-bedroom apartment inside the retirement complex, but eventually Clara required specialized help. The physical separation from his wife hit Ken hard—they had been together for over sixty years.

In the beginning of Clara's stay at the memory care facility, Ken visited her four times a week. But for the past few months, he had needed to cut back on his visits.

"I'm running out of gas. It's a real big deal to make it up the hill," he told me during one of our talks, gesturing to the slope between his patio and the parking lot.

Ken no longer drove, but he let his caregiver, Sophie, chauffeur him in his old Toyota Camry so he could go see Clara. Sophie had recently procured a wheelchair for Ken, but he hadn't wanted to use it yet. "I hate to have to be wheeled in there to see Clara. So I tough it out, but geez, it's getting tougher and tougher."

Ken couldn't be sure if his wife recognized him anymore.

"She's getting really, really bad. It's getting iffy now if she even knows me when I go over to visit. But I still go."

By the time Ken went for his final visit a few days after his ninetieth birthday, Clara's Alzheimer's had long made her unable to process or communicate information, so there wasn't much in the way of a formal goodbye. But Ken believed that Clara would have supported his decision to hasten his death. When they were younger, they'd had many philosophical talks about their end-of-life wishes. Ken was convinced that he had his wife's blessing.

As I greeted his family, Martin, Derianna, and Ken huddled to go over some last-minute logistics. I could tell that something was off. Ken's voice sounded hoarser than usual and a look of panic flared in his eyes. Martin hadn't remembered that Ken had a pacemaker until just now. He thought it would be safer to turn it off prior to Ken's death to prevent it from jolting him back to life after his heart stopped beating.

Turning off a pacemaker falls under the responsibility of a cardiologist, which meant that Ken would have to postpone his death. Martin stepped into the bedroom to make some calls.

Ken chastised himself. He had been so careful to put all the pieces in place. Two days ago, he had called Derianna late at night to ask if he should still take his heart medications on the day of his death. He didn't need to, she had said. He also wanted to know which foods to avoid to maximize his body's absorption of the lethal dose. "Nothing too fatty," she had advised, so no steak the night before. And now this.

Minutes later, Martin reemerged with the good news: the pacemaker could remain on. Unlike other pacemakers, Ken's didn't have a defibrillator, so it wouldn't interfere with his plan to die. Ken heaved a sigh of relief and lowered his tall frame into his armchair. His dog Fluffy, a white shih tzu, jumped onto his lap. Smiling broadly, Ken folded his veiny hands around her. He locked eyes with Martin, who nodded and stepped closer.

Kneeling in front of Ken so they could be at eye level, Martin held a bottle of Seconal, a powerful barbiturate, between his thumb and index finger. It had Ken's first and last name written on the label.

"Do you know what this medication will do to you, Ken?" Martin asked. The question was part of a protocol the doctor followed each time to ensure that a patient fully grasped what was about to happen.

Ken lifted his eyebrows and puckered his lips. He was gearing up for a joke. At the last moment, he thought better of it. Ken sat up straight.

"I will never wake up again."

"Do you still want to proceed?" Martin needed to know.

Ken couldn't resist.

"Well, I wouldn't want to chicken out now. The party's already in full swing and all the guests are here."

Martin rested his mocha eyes on Ken, waiting patiently, studying his face. There was a tenderness in the doctor's mannerisms that surprised me every time I saw him interact with a patient. What I had initially mistaken as shy reserve was a deep and abiding empathy for human hardship. I sometimes wondered if he had chosen medicine or if medicine had chosen him. Martin told Ken that it wasn't too late for him to change his mind. They could call the whole thing off right now, Martin said evenly.

A sense of alarm flashed across Ken's face.

"No, I want to go through with it," Ken said, holding the doctor's gaze. He sounded more sincere now, more resolute.

Their exchange reminded me of a similar conversation I had with Ken about a month ago. I had asked him if he thought he might change his mind when it came closer to the end. He had stared at me with a firmness I had never seen in him before.

"No! Not me. If we're gonna rob a bank, we're gonna rob a bank, OK?"

At the time, I broke into a grin and thought, *I would rob a bank with you.* I liked Ken. Some people probably found his sense of humor grating, but to me his candor felt refreshing. Even at ninety, Ken didn't let anyone put him over a barrel. But he also knew that not everyone shared his sense of relief that his life would soon be over.

"I have to respect the kids too," he had said to me. "I don't want to try to make a happy occasion out of what they think is a sad occasion. But I think they're realistic about it."

Ken's sons knew about their father's daily physical struggles. How numbness crept up his arms. How fluid retention caused his limbs to inflate. How he had started urinating blood. How every time he exerted himself, he would experience a piercing pain in his chest. How he could barely walk the fifty feet to the parking lot outside his back door—even with the assistance of a walker and Sophie's help—without feeling like he was having a heart attack.

"I'm getting worse every day," he had told me, the weary look in his eyes amplified by his droopy eyelids and tinted glasses. "I don't want to have a stroke and have the boys take care of me and my wife. I'm more afraid of living than I am of dying."

Ken had experienced a few close calls in his life. In high school, he and five of his friends drove off a seaside cliff in a 1941 Plymouth, totaling the car but escaping unharmed. The Santa Cruz paper called it "The St. Patrick's Day Miracle." When he was forty, Ken crashed again. This time, he lost control of his car as he flew around a corner, spun in a circle, and skidded off the road. Hanging on to the steering wheel, he remembered thinking, *This time you've had it, you son of a bitch.* Then, a split second later, *No, goddamn it. You're gonna make it.* Ken hit a tree. The impact drove the engine right onto the seat next to him. With gas dripping onto his seat, he climbed out of the wreckage and crawled up the embankment with a broken foot and set of cracked ribs. Eventually, he caught a ride with some highway patrol officers.

Then, about twelve years ago, Ken became almost totally immobilized by stenosis in his neck. Unable to walk or feel his limbs and struggling just to breathe, he was transported to a hospital in Southern California. A specialist told him that it might be too late for surgery. Ken glared at him and said, "Kill me or cure me. No in between."

Ken spent eight and a half hours in the operating theater, and the surgery was declared a success. But he got little reprieve, because soon after, he was diagnosed with colon cancer. The doctor removed six feet of his gut—Ken liked to joke that, to this day, he had no idea what they did with it. The pacemaker came shortly afterward.

At ninety, Ken knew his luck was running out. He suffered from congestive heart failure, a leaky heart valve, and an aggressive form of prostate cancer. Five months before I met Ken, his primary care physician had finally enrolled him in home hospice care.

When Ken told his oldest son, Zack, that he intended to use Oregon's assisted dying law, Zack expressed his support.

"My feeling is that Western medicine has kept Dad alive years past when he would have naturally died," Zack later told me. "If he stopped all the pills that keep him going and had his pacemaker removed, he would be gone within a week. That's no different than saying, 'I'm going to speed it along by taking something to do it.' The end result is the same."

Besides his deteriorating health, Ken's main problem was that he could no longer do the things that once filled his life with meaning. He spent most of his days sitting in a chair watching TV. He still had songs he could write in his head and paintings he could imagine, but the arthritis in his finger joints deterred him from playing his blues guitar, and it turned painting into an onerous task. He still watched horse races, boxing matches, and golf tournaments, but he didn't care who won anymore. His laundry list of maladies had turned living into a chore, stealing all pleasure and purpose from the days he had left.

"The kids are all raised and all off," he said during one of our visits, pointing to the framed pictures of his sons, their wives, and their children, who posed for yearly photographs with their toothy smiles in front of sky-blue canvasses. "I love seeing my grandchildren. I see them once a week, but that isn't an excuse for hanging around either."

His son Tony had recently offered to have Ken move in with him to be closer to the kids, but Ken had declined. He could handle being around his grandkids for only an hour at a time; he just didn't have the energy anymore. Instead, he and Tony had taken a ride around a nearby city park to find a spot for spreading his cremated ashes.

"You've been working on surviving all your life," Ken went on. "You're always trying to get a better house, better clothes, better food, a better car, go to a better movie. You're always thinking about improving yourself and living better. And then, all of a sudden, none of that means anything anymore."

Ken paused, coughing up some phlegm and catching his breath.

"If it weren't for modern medicine, none of these old fogies would be here," he said, tipping his head toward the hallway that led to the other apartments. "They're all hanging on to life like it's something really worth hanging on to, and it isn't really all that."

———————

In Ken's living room, Martin reached into a paper bag from the pharmacy to retrieve Ken's premedications, pills that would settle his stomach and prevent nausea and anxiety once he took the lethal dose of Seconal. The premedications typically take an hour to go into effect. In many ways, they start the clock on an assisted death—physically as much as logistically. Martin unscrewed the two bottles and handed Ken one pill of Zofran and two pills of Reglan. The clock read 10:50 a.m.

Ken reclined in his armchair, looking satisfied. He and his family started reminiscing about his irreverent past: about the fortunes he made and lost in the San Francisco real estate business; his car wash business that prospered and tanked; the thirty-two cars he had owned in his life; his rambunctious, early days as a blues musician; the women he chased before settling down with Clara; the house he built with his own hands. His audience indulged him, reveling with Ken in the soft glow of a bygone era.

"You had a darn good run, Dad," said Zack. "You taught both of us to be hard workers." Ken beamed. He'd had a full life. He had told me so many times himself.

Derianna and I retreated into the kitchen for one of the more tedious tasks that morning—preparing Ken's medication. It goes twice as fast with two people, she said, and I didn't mind having something practical to do. Though families are perfectly capable of opening the capsules, Derianna liked to spare them the task. After all, it is one thing to support a loved one's decision to die and another to physically assemble their fatal cocktail. I pulled up a chair across the table from her.

Derianna popped the lid off Ken's Seconal bottle and showed me what to do: twist open a capsule, dump the powder into a bowl, and sweep out the remaining morsels with the brush head of a special plastic toothpick—from the Dollar Tree, she said.

Prying apart the first few capsules, I couldn't keep my hands from shaking. Here we were, readying the concoction that would end Ken's life while he was chatting away in the next room. I felt a heady sense of transgression rise up inside me. I had never helped anyone die before. Derianna had done it dozens of times. At seventy-seven, she was the oldest and longest serving assisted dying volunteer in Oregon, riding across the state and neighboring Washington in her silver Prius to be with patients in their final hours.

A former nurse and midwife, Derianna treated a death the same way she treated a birth—as a sacred transition from one state of being to another. Her job, as she saw it, was to help facilitate that transition and carry a person over the threshold between life and death.

"You're going to the gate with them and you are letting them go, but you're nurturing them through the gate," she once told me.

Recalling her words now, the shaking stopped and I settled into the work, twisting and pouring in silence. Half an hour later, the task was complete: one hundred orange pill carcasses sat in one bowl, the small mound of white powder in another. We scrubbed our hands at the kitchen sink. An ornate plaque hung over the sink read: "Martha Stewart doesn't live here." Derianna and I stifled a snicker.

Ken's voice boomed from across the living room. He was basking in memories of his great-grandchildren. "They are cuter than a bug," he called out. He proceeded to divide up the paintings on his walls, assigning who would get each of them when he was gone.

Then he addressed me and Derianna, raising his voice a few more decibels.

"By the way, take all the booze in the fridge that you want. And make sure you clean this place up after I'm gone!"

Derianna let out a chuckle, her short gray curls shaking with delight.

Despite Ken's bravado, I knew that he felt a sense of trepidation about his looming departure. He had once admitted as much. "I think anybody would be apprehensive about going to the 'undiscovered country from whose woods no traveler returns,'" he had said to me, quoting Shakespeare. "If you're planning it and you know it, it's spooky. I guess it would be spookier for someone who is a believer."

Ken had always been a staunch atheist. Though he and Sophie didn't see eye to eye on spiritual matters, she would sometimes talk to him about her belief in God and the afterlife—to no avail.

"I don't know what you believe," Sophie told me privately, "but I am very concerned about his soul."

Ken didn't share her concerns. But that didn't mean he was unaware of the gravity of his plan. "I'm trying to visualize a world without me," he said during our final visit before his death, pensive and serious. I thought I heard a hint of melancholy in his voice.

On the morning of his death, you wouldn't have been able to detect any of that. Ever the gracious host, Ken kept offering his guests food and drink when lulls threatened to puncture the conversation. He had wanted to make sure there would be enough cheese and crackers at his gathering, so guests could transition directly into the wake—a joke that cracked him up even as he was telling it. Now, he pulled out another.

"When they put me into the body bag, make sure they leave a little space for my finger just in case I need to unzip it again."

"Don't worry, Dad. We will put a bell in there with you," Zack said and winked.

In the kitchen, Derianna transferred the medication into a wine glass and pulled a tiny whisk from a ziplock bag. She ran water into the glass—first the hot and then the cold to properly dissolve the powder and prevent any clumping. When she was done stirring, she motioned for me to try the cocktail. She knew I'd been curious about Seconal, which had a reputation for being terribly bitter. The families I met during my research frequently mentioned this fact, expressing frustration that the final taste of life was so unpleasant.

I scraped my index finger along the whisk and stuck it into my mouth. The drops tasted so revolting, every bud on my tongue recoiled in disgust. If someone had distilled the essence of bitter, this would be it. I scrambled for a chaser.

Derianna threw me a sympathetic glance.

"No one would ever drink this unless they had to," she said.

Derianna and her colleagues had been trying to find ways to reduce the bitterness of the medication by mixing the powder into sweet juices or having patients chase it down with hard liquor. The latest idea was to have them swish around a flat Coke in their mouth after drinking the lethal dose. I tried some of the Coke Derianna had brought for that purpose. It didn't help very much. Hours later, the vile taste of Seconal would linger in my mouth.

Ken, still reigning in his armchair, fiddled with his iPhone and sent out a few messages. I was struck by the finality and simultaneous banality of the moment: something as commonplace as typing up a text message takes on a much different meaning when you know it'll be your last contact with someone. That was the thing about Ken's death. It felt both momentous and strangely mundane. Even in the midst of a death, people get hungry, use the bathroom, and scroll through their phones. Yet everyone knows that something extraordinary is about to take place.

Ken put his phone down and looked at Martin. It was 11:45 a.m. Almost time.

———

Ken announced that he was going for a leak, rose unsteadily to his feet, and bumped his walker across the carpet. A few minutes later, he emerged and shuffled into the bedroom. He asked his granddaughter to join him so they could have a private moment together. Minutes later, he called for the rest of us.

Seated on the edge of his bed, feet touching the floor, Ken requested that his family flank him on either side. Martin, Derianna, Sophie, and I stood in a cluster near the doorway. I rested my back against one of the bedroom walls, thankful for the extra support.

Tony cued up the song Ken had chosen to accompany his death—"Nothin' about the Blues"—written and performed by Ken himself, with the help of his sons.

"That record really signifies a lot of stages of my life," Ken had told me when he gave me a copy of the album a month prior. "It really shows you what kind of a life I lived, and it's nothing to be proud of, OK? But it was exciting."

At Ken's bidding, Derianna handed him the wine glass with the lethal medication. It looked thick and milky, a dense paste pierced by a wide, stocky straw to help transport it to the back of the mouth quickly, bypassing some of the taste receptors for bitterness. But Ken didn't want to use a straw. Derianna wasn't surprised. In her experience, a lot of men refused straws—they found them degrading, unmanly somehow.

The moment he heard the first few notes of his song blasting from the speakers, Ken lifted the drink to his lips and swallowed the contents. The bitterness didn't faze him at all. When he was done, Derianna offered him some Coke, spiked with Fireball, per his request. Gulping it down, he wiped his lips with the back of his hand and handed the empty glass back to her.

I could feel the back of my throat constrict. Ken had said he wanted to be gone by noon. He looked at his watch. It was 11:52 a.m. The music kept playing.

"Don't care if I win or I looooose," Ken crooned to the sound of his own voice, his live baritone only slightly overpowering the one booming from the record. "I don't know nothin' about the blues."

And then it all happened very fast. As Ken began reciting his epitaph, his words slurred and trailed off:

Walking on eggshells
Hanging by a thread
Not really living
Not really dead
I'm all used up
Nothing left to give
All my time is spent
Just trying to live
That's why I've chosen
Not to be
And let the world turn
Minus me

Ken closed his eyes, his head dropping low on his chest, and drifted off to sleep. Tony and Zack removed his shoes and lifted his legs onto the bed so he could rest comfortably on his side. His dog nestled in the nook between Ken's thighs and his belly. Ken's sons formed a circle around his granddaughter and held each other, weeping.

I felt tears burning in my eyes, but I didn't want to cry in front of the family. I was glad when Derianna motioned for me to join her, Sophie, and Martin in the living room. Hands in our pockets, we stood around, chatting quietly, keeping an eye on the clock. Now all there was to do was wait.

I could see why the idea of being in charge of your death appealed to people who had always run their own show. Ken was one of them. A week ago, he had told me how tickled he felt that he would cheat his facility out of their rent for June—he planned to die just a few days before the end of May, on Memorial Day. Blinking through the tears, I cracked a smile. I felt happy for Ken. It looked like he had succeeded in having the death he desired. I would miss our conversations, but I knew that even without taking his death into his own hands, he wouldn't have stuck around for very much longer.

Ten minutes later, Martin stepped back into the bedroom, and Derianna and I followed. Ken's skin had turned ashen already; his jaw was slightly open. The doctor bent over Ken's torso and listened for a heartbeat with his stethoscope. He felt for Ken's pulse at his neck. He put his hand on his chest. Then he looked up at the bedroom clock, which read 12:08 p.m.

"He's gone," said Martin, his voice on the edge of breaking.

Everyone filed out of the room, except Fluffy, who remained pressed up against Ken's lifeless body.

Once the fact of Ken's death had sunken in, Tony and Zack approached Martin and Derianna to thank them for enabling Ken to die the way he wanted. They were surprised at how quickly Ken went.

"He was determined and ready to go," Derianna told the family, squeezing their hands. She said they could take as much time as they needed before notifying hospice of Ken's passing. His hospice nurses had known of Ken's plan all along.

Sophie, who had agreed to adopt Fluffy, helped Derianna and me gather Ken's prescription medications—there were about twenty bottles. The three of us emptied them into a half-gallon ziplock bag. Derianna added wet coffee grounds to render the drugs unusable before tossing the bag into the garbage. Ken's hospice nurses would have done the very same thing, but she wanted to save them some time.

Zack joined us in the kitchen. He said how grateful he felt for the chance to say goodbye to his dad. For the previous few months, Zack had grown nervous every time an unexpected call came in, fearing that his father had suddenly died. Being able to ready himself for Ken's death—knowing when and how he was planning to die—allowed Zack to be more intentional about how he wanted to leave things with his dad. The day before, Zack had had a long talk with him.

"I got to say everything that needed saying. I told him that I loved him and that I cared for him. And that I appreciated all the things he had done raising me."

Zack just hadn't been sure how to prepare for Ken's death logistically. To do something, he had purchased an impressive quantity of sandwiches, which sat untouched in the fridge.

"It's hard to know what's appropriate," he said.

I nodded, recalling my struggle to choose an outfit for the day. It was, indeed, hard to know what's appropriate.

After bidding Ken's family and Sophie goodbye, Martin, Derianna, and I walked back to the front desk to sign out of the guest log. This part never ceased to feel strange to me. In the space between the two timestamps on the sign-in sheet, a person had died.

The three of us stepped out into the warm midday sun. We didn't talk much. But before we parted ways, Derianna shared her feelings about the death we had just witnessed.

"Ken sung himself out," she said and smiled.

A New Way to Die

When Ken took his leave from this world, he gathered around him family and friends, and he curated his own departure. Though he felt wistful for the people he would leave behind, Ken knew that his days were numbered, and he turned toward death with a sense of relief.

For much of American history, the idea of carefully choosing the terms of your own death would have been unthinkable and is perhaps still unthinkable for some today. In a culture in which death has been largely rendered invisible—tucked away in nursing homes, hospitals, and mortuaries—selecting the day you die and inviting people to your death might seem frivolous. Yet at the end of a long line of failed or foregone treatment options, patients whose physicians have designated them as "terminal" must forge their own path forward. In a growing number of states today, that path includes the option of having an assisted death, but it's a path we are only just beginning to examine and understand. *The Day I Die* is about that path—what stands in its way medically, legally, culturally, and emotionally—and why people like Ken pursue it anyway.

Medical assistance in dying offers a legal way for a terminally ill, mentally competent adult patient to end their life by ingesting a lethal medication prescribed by their physician. Patients with serious cognitive impairment, such as advanced dementia, are excluded from assisted dying laws in America, even if they have a terminal prognosis. Assisted dying laws also specify that patients must be able to ingest the life-ending medication themselves—euthanasia, the act of a physician ending a patient's life with a lethal injection, is expressly forbidden.

For over a decade, from 1997 to 2008, Oregon was the only state that permitted a medically assisted death. Since then, nine other states and Washington, DC, have legalized the practice. By July 2021, one in five Americans lived in a state with legal access to assisted dying.[1] The battlefronts are no longer confined to traditionally blue states either. Americans everywhere are increasingly drawn to having a say in how they die. According to a 2018 Gallup poll, seven in ten Americans think that physicians should be able to help terminally ill patients die.[2]

And not just Americans. Across the globe, more countries have moved toward legalizing assisted dying now than at any other time in history. Germany, Italy, Spain, and Portugal have taken decisive steps toward legalization, preparing to join the ranks of New Zealand, Australia (in Victoria and Western Australia), Belgium, the Netherlands, Luxembourg, Canada, Colombia, and Switzerland. Even in predominantly Catholic countries like Spain, public acceptance of assisted dying is on the rise.[3]

In 2018, the year Ken died, assisted dying accounted for just 0.5 percent of all deaths in Oregon.[4] But the practice has drawn outsize public attention. Since the heartrending story of Brittany Maynard—a young woman from California who suffered from an aggressive brain tumor and, in 2014, relocated to Oregon to die—assisted dying has definitively moved into the national spotlight. Major news outlets have run feature stories on assisted dying, local papers publish op-eds on it almost daily, and filmmakers have dedicated several feature films and TV episodes to the topic.[5] If the right to die was relevant before, it is even more so today.

In an effort to capture the full scope of this issue, I spent five years shadowing those on the front lines of assisted dying in America. I wanted to know how access to an assisted death was transforming the ways Americans died. How do patients summon the will to swallow a lethal medication? How do families find it in themselves to honor such a wish, when it means forever losing a loved one? How does the purpose of medicine change when doctors are not only asked to be healers but also to help people die? And why do so many obstacles continue to block the path to an assisted death, twenty plus years into its legalization?

My research took me into the intimate spaces of American living rooms and hospital suites, where patients and their families tried to cut a trail through the confusing maze of end-of-life decisions, weighing the promises of modern medicine against some of its pitfalls. I traveled to courtrooms, public hearings, and state archives across the country, focused specifically on the Pacific Northwest, where assisted dying has been legal the longest. For eight months, I worked as a hospice volunteer and accompanied patients during the final weeks of their lives.

My training as a cultural anthropologist had everything to do with how that research unfolded. Anthropology studies human difference in all its forms—not just in ancient times but in the here and now. True to the immersive methodology of my discipline, I embedded myself in the communities I studied, frequently socializing with people outside formal interview settings to seize the rich messiness of life. Anthropologists try to insert themselves into the lives of the people they study to watch and listen closely, and to do as they do. Unlike many journalists, we include ourselves in our stories and adopt a first-person narrative voice to acknowledge the fact that we rarely witness events impartially. We always and already filter events through our own social conditioning, and sometimes our presence alone changes the very dynamics we observe.

It became clear fairly quickly that I wouldn't be able to study death the same way I had studied other academic topics—keeping the subject at arm's length and stuffing it into a mental drawer at the end of the day. My research consumed me, and it touched me on a deep emotional level. There were times when I would ride my bike home after an interview with a dying patient and be convinced that everyone I passed on the street was riddled with cancer. My bookshelf started to resemble the bereavement section of a library, and I had to stop reading about death right before I went to sleep. Despite my attempts to protect myself emotionally, I once dreamt I took a lethal dose of barbiturates in error, giving me only three minutes to tell my parents I was about to die. As a society, we do so much to uphold the boundary between life and death, and my work was making that line appear unnervingly thin.

But what surprised me most was that the world of assisted dying was neither as sad nor somber as I had feared. Some of the deaths I attended were so uplifting, funny, and beautiful, they made me forget that I was witnessing a death at all. Because how people like Ken chose to die had everything to do with how they had lived—flaunting convention, calling the shots, and finding levity in their sorrow.

———————————

The Day I Die tackles one of the most defining cultural challenges of our time—how to restore dignity and meaning to the dying process in the age of high-tech medicine. Over the past fifty years, access to life-prolonging technology has radically altered how we die. Today, the majority of Americans die in hospitals, often in intensive care units. Many endure the indignities of a protracted death, not realizing—or realizing too late—that the most advanced medical care may only draw out their suffering. As the surgeon Atul Gawande writes in *Being Mortal*, "In the past few decades, medical science has rendered obsolete centuries of experience, tradition, and language about our mortality and created a new difficulty for mankind: how to die."[6]

Assisted dying reframes how we understand the potential of medicine, not as a way to extend life but to ease the process of dying. An assisted death is much larger than swallowing a lethal dose of medication: it changes how we live, how we die, and how we envision our future. Medical assistance in dying introduces new possibilities for human beings to direct the end of their lives. As I sat with people who contemplated their decision and witnessed some of their deaths first-hand, I saw that this ability to anticipate and even choreograph one's death could be very empowering—for the dying and for those who remain behind. Naming a time and place for their death frequently led to patients feeling a renewed sense of control in a situation that had made them feel totally helpless. It allowed them to think about how they wanted to leave things with their loved ones, repair relationships, and plan for a personalized departure. An assisted death often resulted in less complicated grief as well. Loved ones didn't feel as blindsided.

Yet it isn't as though someone can simply wake up one day and choose to die. America has the strictest assisted dying laws in the world. The country's first law, Oregon's Death with Dignity Act, emerged at the end of a contentious, century-long struggle to legalize some form of medical assistance in dying for very sick patients. After failed ballot initiatives in adjacent states, the Oregon statute was crafted in a context of appeasing monumental opposition and carving out small concessions. Since then, nearly every state that has adopted an assisted dying law has followed the strict Oregon model or, in the case of Hawaii, added more constraints. Though these laws may make the process of dying less painful for some, they don't necessarily make it easier. Current assisted dying laws don't help people with some of the most hopeless diseases, and many barriers to access remain. In trying to reclaim some control over the way they die, some patients are being stripped of that control in the process.

An assisted death in America is the path not of least but of most resistance. Those intending to walk it must overcome an array of obstacles and red tape at a time when their health is rapidly failing, and no patient can realize an assisted death on their own. They have to rely on the participation of many others—physicians, pharmacists, hospice nurses, volunteers, family members—willing to sanction, enable, and ultimately share responsibility for their death. Sometimes patients navigate those waters successfully and manage to secure the coveted bottle of life-ending medication; at other times, the opposition they face along the way jeopardizes their entire plan. And sometimes they simply run out of time.

During my research, I encountered people at different phases in this process—some stymied, some triumphant, many somewhere in between. I met patients who spent months going on a wild goose chase to find physicians willing to participate in the law, especially in rural parts of the country where Catholic health systems ran the only hospital in town. Finding a place to die presented another hurdle: many assisted living facilities prohibit the practice under their roof, forcing patients to make alternative arrangements—sometimes at a nearby motel. Some hospices refused to cooperate with a patient's wish to seek an assisted death, leading patients to feel abandoned. And sometimes the medications didn't work. Expecting they would be gone within minutes, some patients have had prolonged or even failed deaths.

This book draws on these experiences and on hundreds of conversations with those who own a stake in this new way to die. It recounts the stories of ordinary Americans who go to extraordinary lengths to be in control of their deaths. If we want to understand what drives someone to take this path and why anyone helps them, we have to lift the curtain on people's real-life experiences with these laws. In doing precisely that, *The Day I Die* advances an urgent conversation on what exactly the role of medicine should be at the end of life.

As of this writing, the jurisdictions that have legalized assisted dying fall on the progressive end of the spectrum: Oregon, Washington, Vermont, California, Colorado, Hawaii, the District of Columbia, New Jersey, Maine, and New Mexico. Montana is the only exception, and observers usually point to the state's libertarian ethos to explain its outlier status. In fact, assisted dying was only *decriminalized* in Montana in the wake of a 2009 court case (*Baxter v. Montana*) brought by a patient who sued for his right to die. The practice hasn't been positively codified into law, which means there are no legal guidelines for how to go about an assisted death.[7] Physicians just won't face prosecution if they prescribe life-ending medication to a patient.

Yet assisted dying is an issue that transcends party lines. When it comes to their death, people's political leanings aren't always a reliable indicator of what they might choose. Their religious leanings can sometimes be a better guide for whether they might pursue an assisted death or not. Linda Ganzini, a now-retired Oregon psychiatrist with decades of experience studying assisted dying, says that most people who use Oregon's Death with Dignity Act tend to not be very religious. She calls them "the single least religious group of any patients." But even here, there are exceptions. While conservative believers may less commonly seek an assisted death, someone may be deeply devout and still want assistance in dying. When people find themselves in the grips of serious illness, most aren't going to leave any tool on the shelf.

Who uses assisted dying laws? Available statistics show that it is mainly older patients who access medical assistance in dying. In Oregon, 81 percent of those who sought an assisted death in 2020 were sixty-five or older, and the vast majority—about two-thirds—had cancer.[8] That same year, 97 percent of decedents were white.[9] Compared to an overall state population that is 75 percent white, patients who chose assisted dying were overrepresented statistically.[10] A look at a more diverse state confirms this trend: though California is only 37 percent white, people who took advantage of the state's End of Life Option Act in 2019 were 87 percent white.[11]

What might account for unequal use of assisted dying laws by people of color? There are several possible explanations. Communities that are used to receiving inferior healthcare and being denied medical services—based in part on lower rates of insurance—are more likely to choose aggressive life-prolonging measures when these are offered.[12] People who have been historically mistreated by the medical establishment are also less likely to trust a physician to have their best interests in mind, especially when it comes to stopping treatment.[13] Studies reveal that rates of Black enrollment in hospice remain relatively low and that Black people have fewer discussions with their physicians about the end of life.[14] When systemic racism continues to haunt medical encounters in communities of color—and when death itself may be the result of deep-seated health inequalities—then an expedited death might not seem very appealing.[15]

But there are other reasons why members of some communities of color aren't keen on pursuing an assisted death. Rates of religiosity are highest among Black and Latino Americans; choosing an assisted death may go directly against the grain of their spiritual faith.[16] Medical decision-making isn't always an individual decision either—in some communities of color, the family steps in to take on end-of-life care and decisions (which also accounts for lower rates of hospice use).[17] And given that resistance to assisted dying often comes from within the family, a patient's private desire to seek an assisted death may have to take a back seat.

Ultimately, it is hard to separate issues of preference from issues of access. In some cases, the wish for an assisted death might be there, but someone may be unaware that the law exists or how to access it. The social and financial capital required to access an assisted death is considerable: federally funded insurance programs like Medicare don't cover the costs of eligibility appointments or life-ending medication.[18] Unless physicians waive their appointment fees or bill for a general end-of-life consultation, these costs alone can be prohibitive. Patients typically also need help navigating the bureaucracy of assisted dying laws, and if they don't know where to turn, they can quickly get stymied.

The Day I Die will stir many viewpoints, and some readers may find its contents unsettling. There are lots of reasons why someone might be opposed to a medically assisted death. Some people disagree with assisted dying on religious grounds, contending that God alone has the power to end human life. Some argue that assisted dying carries an implicit judgment on what kinds of lives are ultimately deemed livable, heightening existing cultural tendencies to value individual control and able bodies. Some physicians say that assisted dying runs counter to their mission to save lives and that palliative care is sufficient to relieve suffering at the end of life. None of these perspectives should be discounted, and many of them feature in this book.

At the same time, there are people who feel that their life belongs to them alone and who want the right to choose the course and timing of their own death—without having their decision impact anybody else's choices. Their perspectives deserve compassion and curiosity, and a basic willingness to consider their position. That doesn't mean that all is well in the world of assisted dying. An assisted death can be flawed and fallible, and things don't always go the way everyone hopes. Being candid about these limitations is critical for improving care for the dying. It's just as critical to highlight the solace and benefits an assisted death can offer patients whose suffering has melted away any desire to live.

One thing is true: an assisted death is not the easy way out. Hastening the end of your life is an act of will that demands improbable courage. It means accepting the hard truth of your mortality and walking toward death with clear, open eyes.

PART I

Losing Control

CHAPTER 1

Spinning Away

Covering the walls in Joe's home office in Vancouver, Washington, were dozens of glossy medals and framed pictures of running meets—a shrine to the hours and days he had spent pushing himself to the crest of physical triumph. Each of them carried vivid memories of carbo-loading dinners, auspicious bib numbers, and sports drinks in all colors of the rainbow. Now they served as blunt reminders of the life he once had, prediagnosis, when the muscles in his body still stretched, lunged, and churned without special effort, or even thought.

One of the photos shows Joe, probably in his late forties, in dark-blue shorts and a bright-yellow T-shirt. His short hair hemmed in by a white headband, he wears aviator sunglasses and a look of concentration on his face as he sprints the last couple of miles toward the finish line of the Portland marathon. The course flattens out here as runners weave their way through the downtown area to a shrill chorus of bystanders. Right behind Joe, a younger man with wiry legs picks up the chase. But

Joe stares straight ahead and his stride looks strong. It's clear that he won't go down without a fight.

By the time I met Joe on a Sunday morning in early 2018, the days of his physical feats were long gone. As I walked up to greet him, he lay immobile in the middle of his living room in a dark leather recliner. A brown duvet was pulled up to his neck, warming a body that wouldn't obey him anymore. Solemn and alert, Joe's denim-blue eyes peered out at me from behind his round, metal-rimmed glasses. Behind him, the rain drummed on a sliding glass door that opened into a drenched backyard. The rain wasn't unusual for this time of year, late February in the Pacific Northwest, but it added a brittle layer of gloom to the space.

When I had called his partner, Anna, to arrange the visit, she immediately launched into a description of all the roadblocks she and Joe had been facing to qualify him for Washington's assisted dying law. She was talking fast, like a person frustrated by an unmet desire to be heard. I knew from my research with other families that navigating the bureaucracy of assisted dying laws could be a full-time job. But I was surprised to learn that someone with a clear-cut terminal diagnosis was having such difficulty.

In September 2016, at age seventy-two, Joe was diagnosed with ALS—amyotrophic lateral sclerosis, also known as Lou Gehrig's disease—a progressive neurological disorder that destroys neurons responsible for muscle movement. In the United States, about six thousand people are diagnosed with ALS every year, and the disease's etiology still remains largely a mystery. After the initial onset of symptoms, the average life expectancy ranges from two to five years as the body's muscle groups shut down one by one.

Joe was polite and soft-spoken. His lopsided smile, encased by a closely trimmed snow-white beard, surfaced only occasionally, when something truly amused him. Half an hour into our conversation, as I asked Joe and Anna to reconstruct the events of the past year and a half, Joe broke into a metallic cough. He motioned his chin toward the glass of water that sat between him and Anna on a side table.

"His mouth has felt exceptionally dry today," Anna offered by way of an explanation. She picked up the glass and held it for him, waiting for his tongue to catch the straw.

"I think I may have to have a manual cough assist," Joe whispered, his voice grainy and barely audible. Anna rose to her feet.

"With ALS, you lose your core strength, your diaphragm, which you need for coughing," Anna said as she peeled the duvet from Joe's body, baring his pale arms and legs, which had lost nearly all muscle definition. "So we have a machine to clear the mucus in his airway, but Joe has discovered that this little thing we do is actually more effective."

Anna removed his head and neck rests and pressed a button on his recliner. Joe's body slid slowly down and out of the chair. When his furry moccasin slippers hit the ground, she hoisted him up—he could still stand, but his upper body was so limp that he almost toppled over— and scooped him up from behind. Though Anna was much smaller than Joe, she didn't seem to be straining. Joe was thin as a wafer.

Joe hung in Anna's arms like a rag doll—his head drooping low on his chest, shoulders perched forward, and arms sagging by his sides like two power lines cut down by a storm. He used to be a tall man, but the disease had compressed his spinal cord.

Anna tightened her embrace and folded her hands flat on top of each other underneath his rib cage. "Ready?" she asked.

Joe murmured his response, looking straight down. On the count of three, Anna dug her hands into his abdomen in a quick upward motion while Joe tried to clear his throat. A feeble sound emerged. She pressed in again. Again.

"It takes timing but, you know, we're dancers. We've got timing," she said, shooting me an apologetic glance. I told her that I didn't mind, wishing she could forget about me for a second, a witness to their tragic dance.

The fourth time, Joe emitted a forceful, guttural cough. "That was a good one," Anna said, carefully releasing her embrace and helping Joe sink back into his recliner. He was still looking down, his neck muscles no longer strong enough to keep his head upright.

"You can see, this is just a laugh a minute, isn't it?" Anna said, trying to diffuse the lingering intimacy between us. She tucked her straight, silver hair behind her ears and stole a quick glance at Joe. He cracked a smile, fleeting but just in time for her to catch it.

Anna settled Joe back into the chair, propping his head up with two pillows and his neck brace. She knew exactly how to arrange everything. You could tell she had done it a hundred times. The whole ordeal had made Joe thirsty, and he had her lift the glass of water to his lips again so he could bite down on the straw. Joe closed his eyes. For a second, I wondered if he was going to drift off to sleep, but then he opened them again and looked at me, ready for the next question.

In the midsummer of 2016, Joe noticed weakness in his left hand during his weekly pickleball game. Pickleball combines elements of badminton, tennis, and table tennis. Players wield wooden or composite paddles on a small court. Joe was right-handed, but he couldn't get a good grip anymore when he used his left hand to pick up the ball. At first, Joe suspected that his watch was pressing down on his wrist, perhaps cutting off circulation to his hand. When the weakness persisted after playing without his watch, he thought he had strained his wrist or slept on it wrong. *Maybe a pinched nerve*, he speculated. But when the sensation didn't go away weeks later, he went to see a neurologist.

Anna was standing in the kitchen when Joe returned from his appointment. She had no reason to feel alarmed. She thought he was going to tell her that they had scheduled an MRI or X-ray for him. But he had other news for her.

"Everybody has to die some time," Joe said.

"What?" Anna felt the ground turn unsteady beneath her feet.

"The doctor is pretty sure, in fact, he's certain, that I have ALS."

Joe understood that ALS was fatal, but he didn't have any idea of how the disease would progress. His neurologist hadn't gone into much detail with him that day.

Anna clutched the counter and burst into tears. She knew exactly what an ALS diagnosis meant. One of her elementary school friends, a dentist, had died of ALS in his late thirties. She knew that ALS led to paralysis and went from one part of the body to another while the brain remained completely active—"a cruel joke," she called it.

Tom Samuels, one of the specialists Joe started seeing months later, had long studied the unique challenges an ALS diagnosis brings. A pulmonologist from Portland, Samuels wasn't licensed in Washington, but Joe's health plan allowed him to see doctors within the Providence healthcare system across the Columbia River in Oregon. When I met Samuels at a coffee shop in Portland, he explained that ALS impacts three different groups of muscles.

"ALS affects the extremities, so arms and legs," he said. "In about two-thirds of patients, that's the first thing they notice. They may get a little foot drop or weakness in one hand that progresses. About a third of all patients, the first thing that goes is their speech and the ability to swallow. It's called bulbar onset. Then, about one percent of patients, the first thing they notice is shortness of breath, because the breathing muscles become affected."

"But everyone eventually gets everything," he added. "If they live long enough."

I asked Samuels what patients with ALS eventually die from.

"Ninety-nine percent die from respiratory failure," he said. "The breathing muscles get so weak that they can't get carbon dioxide out. So the carbon dioxide builds up. The good news about that is that carbon dioxide acts like morphine on the brain—it basically puts the brain to sleep. It's usually not a sudden episode; they usually have a buildup, lapse into a coma, and then they die. But occasionally people will choke to death. It's a miserable way to die."

Samuels's explanation made me see Anna's Heimlich maneuver in a new light. Had Joe been terrified of choking to death the morning I met him? If most patients with ALS could expect a death from respiratory failure, as Samuels suggested they did, then running out the clock on an ALS diagnosis didn't seem like an especially comforting option.

For the first couple of months after his diagnosis, Anna and Joe floated about their weeks in a daze, partially in denial, partially in fear of what lay ahead. Neither of them felt ready to face the full weight of Joe's diagnosis. Initially, Anna and Joe didn't talk much about what it would all mean—it was just too painful. They didn't put up a tree for Christmas that year, but they still showed up to their weekly contra dances, and Joe continued with pickleball and his Zumba classes, a dance he had discovered only months before.

Joe met Anna contra dancing in 2010. She was living in Tacoma after her divorce when she attended a daylong contra dance in Portland. Joe, who had been married twice before, immediately noticed her on the dance floor. He felt too shy to properly introduce himself, but he asked her to dance five waltzes that night. They were together from then on. Anna moved into the house in Vancouver Joe had bought after his retirement as a software engineer, and they began making a home together.

In their desire to prolong the amount of time they would have to enjoy dancing together, Joe and Anna soon became obsessed with finding possible treatments. Right on the heels of their early refusal to engage with Joe's news came a period of intense bargaining.

"We reached out in a million different directions. What are the treatments? Who's doing what research?" Anna recalled. "Can you go to Japan for a clinical trial? Can you do this? Can you do that?"

They compiled a stack of notes on various kinds of treatment and lugged it with them to Joe's next appointment at the ALS clinic.

"And we could tell when we brought up all these things that seemed promising to us that they really weren't," said Anna. Joe's neurologist suggested some trials Joe might consider, but he would have had to come into the clinic every day to receive infusions.

"It would have basically taken up his whole life," Anna went on, "and all they can do is slow down your progression. And if you're too far along and you've lost too many abilities, they don't want to slow your progression down because they don't want to arrest you in this bad condition. It's not like with cancer where you have different kinds of chemotherapy and radiation. With ALS, it's just a downward spiral. It's just a matter of how fast it's going to be."

In a society that trades in military metaphors when talking about illness—when cancer patients become "warriors" and "survivors" and cells foreign "invaders"—the idea of foregoing even the sliver of a chance for more time can feel like premature surrender. After all, the next miracle cure could be just around the corner, the next experimental drug one clinical trial away.

"Abuse of the military metaphor may be inevitable in a capitalist society," writes Susan Sontag. "War-making is one of the few activities that people are not supposed to view 'realistically'; that is, with an eye to expense and practical outcome. In all-out war, expenditure is all-out, unprudent—war being defined as an emergency in which no sacrifice is excessive."[1]

Turning your back on the powerful cultural machinery of life extension can feel like trying to swim upstream. That's why some assisted dying patients struggle with being perceived as "quitters" when they push back against the ubiquitous logic that more time is always better. The decision to stop "fighting" to reclaim what life someone is able to have here and now almost amounts to an act of conscientious objection.

For his part, Joe had no intention of running the full gamut of what ALS held in store for him: the air hunger that would only get worse and the prospect of becoming "locked in"—when he would no longer be able to move or speak or swallow but would remain mentally alert. Joe's initial frustration over not having any viable treatment options soon gave way to a decision. He wouldn't let this brutal disease get the best of him, only waiting for the other shoe to drop—not if he could help it. He would be the one to decide when and how he was going to die.

He would hasten the end of his life.

In America, an incurable medical condition alone isn't enough to qualify someone for assistance in dying—a patient must also be within imminent reach of their death. By the time a patient is approved for an assisted death, they must already be within six months of the end of their life, coinciding with the admission criteria for hospice. Open-ended prognoses that are typical for painful, protracted degenerative diseases like ALS don't fulfill this condition for terminality, at least not until a patient's breathing becomes severely compromised.

Physicians in Washington and Oregon usually won't give ALS patients the required six-month prognosis until it is clear that their lung capacity has measurably deteriorated. Specialists like Samuels perform a variety of tests that assess lung function to determine if a patient is nearing the six-month mark. One of these exams is called a vital capacity test.

"You take the deepest breath you can and blow it out all the way to the bottom," Samuels explained. "And that's your vital capacity. And roughly, an adult woman is about four liters and an adult man is about five liters, depending on height and age. When someone is diagnosed for ALS, they take that breathing test. And when their vital capacity gets down below fifty percent of what it was at diagnosis, we know they're getting close to dying. And it depends on how soon they get there. If they're at one hundred percent in January and by June they're at fifty percent, they're not going to make it to the end of the year. But if they're at one hundred percent in 2012 and at seventy-five percent in 2018, they've got a long way to go."

Yet by the time a patient becomes eligible for an assisted death on account of their now-limited life span, they may have missed the window in which they can self-administer the lethal medication—a cornerstone of assisted dying laws in America. The physical manifestations of many advanced neurodegenerative diseases like ALS bump up against this rule. Alongside their diminishing ability to breathe, patients with ALS almost always lose their ability to swallow. If a patient can no longer swallow, they may choose to receive the drugs another way. That's because physicians have interpreted the concept of ingestion to mean any method that involves a person's digestive system. In addition to taking the medications orally, patients can ingest them through a feeding tube or a rectal catheter—as long as *they* are the ones pushing down on the syringe.

There's just one problem: squeezing a syringe poses a nearly impossible challenge for patients like Joe who have lost the use of their hands.

Anna was upset that Joe would be expected to administer his own death. To her, the rule felt both arbitrary and punitive.

"Why do they make people self-administer?" Anna asked me. "You can verify that somebody wants it. Why do you make them do it themselves? The act of it, there's the will, the wanting it to be over. Wanting to go to sleep and not wake up, because of what *happens* when you wake up. What if Joe lost his ability to swallow? He could wake up one morning and not have it. And then he would be sunk."

Samuels had a similar reaction when I asked him about the problem of self-administration.

"The law was not written for ALS," he told me. "You have to be able to ingest the medication yourself. And here you have got all these patients who can't even swallow."

Patients, doctors, and families jump through fantastical hoops to make sure they adhere to the self-administration guidelines imposed by assisted dying laws. For instance, a patient who can no longer swallow but still has limited finger movement can have their feeding tube adjusted in such a way that they pull on a tiny rubber band or remove a clip that delivers the medication through the tube. Some patients release the plunger with the side of their head. Others use the remaining dexterity of one finger to push the lever on their wheelchair and ram it into the wall at such an angle that it presses the syringe on their feeding tube. The point is that a patient must be able to start and stop the flow of medication on their own. That action, however tiny, is seen as expressing a prized American value—autonomous will—a final safeguard meant to ensure the voluntary nature of a patient's death.

Charles Blanke, an oncologist with years of experience prescribing medications under Oregon's assisted dying law, became furious every time he raised the example of the wheelchair.

"To say that an ALS patient has to be able to ram their wheelchair into a wall—come on. Is that really different than having their son, with their wishes being clearly known, push the syringe? Obviously, it's different for the son, but is it different for the patient?"

Blanke criticized the fact that patients who were too sick to self-administer the lethal drugs were excluded from using the law altogether.

"And there are lots of them," he said. "It's discriminatory."

The stress over their ability to swallow can provoke a great deal of anxiety in patients, particularly when it comes to correctly timing their exit. Doing it too early means cutting short a life still worth living; waiting too long means they might miss their chance. Aware of their ever-shrinking window to use the law at all, many assisted dying patients in America choose to die earlier than they otherwise would have liked.

Because Joe wasn't sure if his ability to swallow would hold out long enough for him to use Washington's Death with Dignity law, he wanted a plan in place that would give him an out if his condition became insufferable. That is why, after the initial shock of his diagnosis had set in, Joe began researching Dignitas, a right-to-die organization that facilitates assisted deaths for foreign and Swiss nationals in Switzerland. Joe contacted Dignitas and paid $240 to become a member, a requirement for being able to use their services. The actual cost for an accompanied death through Dignitas is much higher. It starts at $8,000, which covers administrative expenses, a physician's consultation, and the fee for completing an assisted death. What attracted Joe to Dignitas was that he wouldn't have to wait until he qualified for Washington's restrictive law. He would be able to set his own timetable.

In January 2017, Joe went public with his diagnosis. He typed up an open letter to his friends and sent it out via email. "My news," the subject line read.

"I have ALS. You may know that ALS is a disease that attacks the nerves and muscles. It is 100% fatal. There is no cure, and treatments to slow it or improve function do not do much. Needless to say, Anna and I are engaged in coming to grips with this news, planning for changes we will have to make, identifying tasks that need to be completed while we can, and figuring out what to do with the time and abilities I have remaining. For now, I hope to continue with the activities I enjoy doing with all of you. If you see me on the dance floor, at pickleball, in Zumba, please interact with me normally, just as you always have. I will have to give these up in time, but there is no reason not to be positive about the pleasures of today. I am happy to have known you and look forward to interacting with you for some time yet."

Below his signature, Joe inserted his personal tagline, set apart by musical notes: "Never sit down while the music is playing."

Joe himself became fiercely opposed to sitting—in a wheelchair. It was his line in the sand. To Joe, accepting the wheelchair was akin to giving up and admitting defeat by a disease that had already robbed him of so much.

But as his symptoms progressed, Joe began tolerating the incremental loss of his bodily functions. He discovered ways to work around his limitations, starting with a knob he had installed on his steering wheel that allowed him to drive his car with one hand. When he could no longer contra dance—he became unable to put his arms out to circle left or right—he switched over to waltz. Joe had always been an excellent lead, and he found that he could guide expertly with one hand, with his left arm hanging by his side or just barely around his partner.

Yet it pained Anna to watch Joe's steady downward progression. "It just made me so sad that this guy who loved to move and loved to dance and loved to drive was going to lose all that," she said. "Pretty soon, he wouldn't be able to dance anymore. Which is all he cared about, really, was dancing. It was breaking down a lot of inhibitions for him. I could just see in front of me where we were heading."

That summer, Joe and Anna traveled to Alaska on a two-week cruise to the Inside Passage. Joe drove the two of them to the hotel where they boarded the tour bus to Vancouver, Canada, the start of the trip.

"When we got on the ship, most of the dining that we were doing was buffet, and I'd get his food and bring it to him, because he only had one hand," Anna remembered. "But he could still drink from a cup. He could still eat with a fork. And, most importantly, he could still raise his glass when we went to happy hour!" She laughed. "So, you know, it was good. It was really a good thing that we went."

After they returned, reality set in hard. With Joe's mobility getting worse, they decided to sell their house and move into one that could accommodate a wheelchair. Finalizing the sale papers in September, Joe could barely sign his name. He could no longer hold a pen with his right hand, so he bought a signature stamp for all official business. Around the same time, he lost his ability to drive. He could no longer play pickleball. He had stopped attending the dances. He couldn't pick up a sandwich or lead a spoon to his mouth. He had lost twenty pounds. His head had sunk low on his chest and his entire upper body stooped forward.

"If he didn't have the back brace on, he and I were eye to eye," Anna recalled. "I'm five foot five and a half, and he's six foot one. He couldn't hold his head up. He couldn't stand up straight. And everything, everything failed at once."

Joe would walk around the house with his torso perched precariously forward, arms dangling limp by his sides. He was still refusing the wheelchair that Anna had procured for him from the ALS clinic.

Around the end of December, Joe's brother Thomas, a retired physical therapist from Portland, visited them. After watching Joe amble down the hall, he took Anna aside and told her that Joe shouldn't be walking anymore.

"If he ever lost his balance and went down, he couldn't break his fall with his hands and arms," he warned her. "If Joe ever fell, he'd fall right on his forehead and crack his skull. You know, that could kill him."

Anna nodded. She was grateful that Joe had never fallen and hurt himself under her watch, but she also knew that Joe's shuffling around the house was a disaster waiting to happen. If he ever did fall, she wouldn't be able to pick him up.

She remembered pleading with him. "Both the physical therapist and your brother say you should not be walking anymore. You gotta stop walking. You're gonna have to start using the wheelchair." To her surprise, Joe didn't put up a fight this time. When I asked her why, Anna shrugged her shoulders. "Frog in the pot. He got used to it."

Like the frog that doesn't jump out of boiling water if it is heated up slowly, Joe was beginning to surrender to his disease. He knew he didn't want to die violently from a fall or a freak accident. Having relinquished a great deal of control over his functional abilities already, he wished to go out on his own terms—voluntarily and when he was ready. So he agreed to stop walking and start using a wheelchair until the time of his choosing would come.

With each of his losses, Joe's line of what he deemed acceptable shifted. Things that used to seem unimaginable gradually became part of Joe's new routine. His home was now crowded with machines that took over most of his bodily functions: a manual and electric wheelchair, a Hoyer lift, his back and neck braces, a suction machine for his excess saliva, an automatic cough assist apparatus, and a BiPAP machine to help with his breathing through a face mask.

Because of Joe's head drop, which was exacerbated by scoliosis in his neck, brushing his teeth had become a nightly challenge. Anna would transfer him into the manual wheelchair that tilted back and hold him there at an angle while she brushed his teeth. With Joe still slanted back, she would insert the suction saliva machine into his mouth so he wouldn't choke on the watery toothpaste. They would sink into bed each night—Joe in his hospital bed, Anna alone in their queen-size bed next to him—exhausted by Joe's bedtime routines. He had a foot pedal attached with duct tape to his bedsheet that he could press with his toes to sound an alarm when he needed to wake Anna in the middle of the night. With the mask of the BiPAP machine covering his face, she would have been unable to hear him call for her.

Although Joe's line in the sand had slowly shifted over the course of fifteen months, he held on to his original plan of hastening the end of his life. He knew that his death was a loose boulder barreling down the mountain toward him. Powerless to stop it, all he could hope for was to preempt it. Joe no longer faced a meaningful decision between life and death but between one kind of death over another.

Yet he was no longer thinking of using the services of Dignitas. The first few months after his diagnosis, when he was mobile, he could still imagine taking on the trouble and expense of flying to Switzerland. But as time went on, Joe became more incapacitated and vulnerable each day. Pretty soon, the practicality and cost of traveling to Zürich, sitting through the two-week waiting period once he arrived, and being in a foreign country for his death sounded much less appealing and feasible. By the time Joe and Anna started looking into Washington's assisted dying law more seriously, he had all but abandoned his plan to fly to Switzerland.

In January 2018, Joe and Anna went to see his neurologist for his three-month checkup. The neurologist said she was ready to recommend him for home hospice care. Admitting a patient to hospice meant that their life expectancy was estimated to be six months or less. The news took Anna and Joe by surprise.

"I don't think anyone expected him to decline as quickly as he did. It was shocking for us," Anna recalled. "Joe and I looked at each other like 'I guess this is it.' Once Joe was told that he was eligible for hospice, he started moving on his application for Death with Dignity. Being eligible for hospice is that magic six-month number."

It wasn't that hospice was unappealing to Joe; he enrolled immediately and investigated his options for comfort care. Staff from Providence, his hospice provider, said they would try their best to manage his panic-stricken episodes and palliate his air hunger. But their assurances weren't enough to give Joe the confidence he needed that he wasn't going to choke to death. He was already beginning to lose his ability to breathe.

"It's inevitable," Joe told me, referring to the progression of his disease. "Why should I go through all this trouble, all the pain, more loss of ability, more loss of time? It's over anyway. Might as well just..."

His voice trailed off. Anna picked up the thread for him.

"When it gets to the point when all his waking hours are just maintaining his body and trying to keep his body alive, keeping his breathing—"

"There's no life left." Joe cut her off and stared up at the ceiling.

A few weeks before I met Joe, he had spelled out his final thoughts—laboriously—with the help of voice recognition software. On the page, he reflects on the theme of mortality in the works of J. R. R. Tolkien, his favorite author. Joe had always been fascinated by the Númenóreans, a famed race that serves as allies of the elves. Unlike the elves—who are immortal in the sense that they stop aging at a certain point in mature middle age and live forever unless they succumb to accident or war—the Númenóreans are squarely mortal. But when they sensed their period of vitality coming to an end, they could choose to give up their lives voluntarily. Rather than coping with their decline, they could elect to die.

"It is a beautiful and noble vision of a life lived under the shadow of mortality, but devoid of the need to live on after having lost the abilities that we think of as making us who we are," Joe wrote.

Joe had lost most of the qualities that made him who he was. He had long identified himself through his physical feats, his dancing, and his ability to command his body. Now an assortment of machines orchestrated each of his movements. Joe couldn't recognize himself anymore in his new cyborg existence. He could still reason and be methodological, but those things weren't enough to sustain him. When illness has taken away as much from a person as it took from Joe, controlling the timing and terms of one's death can bring enormous relief.

Joe wrapped up his thoughts: "Tolkien's books are fantasy. We are not Numenoreans. If we should contract a disease such as ALS, making it clear that the end of life is near and that approaching death in the natural way is going to be very painful and unpleasant, there is no way by sheer force of will to avoid it. Fortunately, if you live in Oregon or Washington, the next best thing is available to you. Kindly and compassionate people are available who can help you make the last choice that you will ever make, but at least you can make it and not have events thrust upon you that you would not choose."

Joe didn't choose any of this; nobody does. But he rested secure in the belief that in the midst of seeing his body quietly slip away from him, he could have a say over how and when he went. He just wasn't prepared for all the hurdles still to come.

CHAPTER 2

When Hospice Isn't Enough

For seriously ill patients like Joe, hospice usually becomes the default option. In fact, some physicians believe that if patients had better access to robust pain control through hospice, there wouldn't be a need for a medically assisted death at all. And yet for Joe, who didn't want to let things run their course, hospice came up short. His hospice providers couldn't assure him that he wasn't going to die a frightening death. Though Joe liked his hospice team, he knew that hospice couldn't give him the one thing he so desperately desired: some sense of agency in a situation that had made him feel utterly powerless.

I learned this lesson firsthand during my time as a hospice volunteer. I had signed up to work for a Portland-area hospice organization to better understand the context in which end-of-life decisions emerge. Two assignments left an especially strong impression on me. The first assignment was with Ella, a spunky, heavyset Black woman in her eighties. She was living in an adult foster home run by an Ethiopian couple on the outskirts of Portland and had just recently enrolled in hospice care. Ella suffered from congestive heart failure, which drove sharp arrows of pain through her chest in unpredictable intervals. But she refused to let her illness take away her weekly bingo outing, the one activity that still made her feel excited about something.

Every Tuesday, I waited for Ella in the parking lot of a Portland community center to escort her to bingo. Decked out in flaming pink lipstick, Ella would scoot down the van ramp in her wheelchair, hollering, "Let's play, sweetheart!" We would buy our bingo booklets and head over to the dining hall, where seniors armed with fanny packs of daubers were setting up their stations and stocking up on sugary snacks to fuel their game.

The moment the first number was called, Ella became all business. She was there to win, not to make friends. She dreamed about buying a new pair of shoes with her winnings, or maybe an elegant blouse. Growing up, money had always been tight. Ella was born in Jackson, Mississippi, the oldest of four children. Her parents moved the family to the Pacific Northwest when she was young, and her father helped build the Grand Coulee Dam and later worked in the shipyards. For twenty years, Ella punched tickets for Greyhound in Sacramento before finding work as a permit coordinator for the city of Portland. Ella had a passion for traveling; she would take off to the Oregon coast at a moment's notice. Over the past ten years, the radius of her trips gradually shrank. Now weekly bingo was as far as she went. And she savored every minute of it, even as she found it increasingly difficult to keep up.

As the game kicked off, the numbers descended on us at lightning speed. Ella could barely scan and stamp her sheet fast enough before it was on to the next number. I tried to keep one eye on my sheet and one on hers, letting her know when she had missed a number or was close to a bingo. I learned quickly that the other players took no prisoners. "Keep it moving," they grumbled whenever we asked to have a number repeated. Swatting their gripes away, Ella retorted with a slight of her own. But shame on the poor soul who mistakenly yelled "bingo"—the glares were devastating. In the weeks we played together, Ella never won. But I think she enjoyed herself.

Ella's decline was rapid. By our fourth outing, her breathing had become strained, the darts in her chest relentless. She begged Leila, the hospice nurse, to let her keep attending bingo. Leila agreed, but the conditions for our trips turned more stringent. For our fifth outing, Ella carried a bag of oral morphine syringes in her purse, and Leila asked me to monitor her pain level constantly. If Ella said her pain was a four or higher (on a scale from one to ten), I was to call hospice. As the bingo numbers rained down on us that day, Ella bit her lips, missing three numbers in a row as she clutched her heart. Panic fluttering in my stomach, I asked for her pain level. "Seven," she blurted out. I jumped on the phone with Leila, who told me to get out Ella's syringes. One by one, her fingers quivering, Ella dispensed the liquid morphine into her mouth. By then, I already knew that we wouldn't be back.

The last time I saw Ella was at the adult foster home. On my way in, I bumped into Leila. "Ella's actively dying," she told me. Her words felt sobering, like ice water on summer skin. I hadn't been prepared for such a rapid turn. For a second, I hesitated. Then I slipped into Ella's room.

She was asleep, heavily sedated by morphine. "To keep her comfortable," Leila had said.

Ella looked much smaller in her bed than she had out in the world. Her jet-black wig had ridden up on her forehead, exposing her thinning gray hair underneath. Ella's scarlet glue-on nails had slid away from their cuticles, a sign of life's quiet insistence from below. I sank into the chair next to her.

I had no idea how Ella felt about what was happening to her. We had never talked about the end of her life. I wanted to believe that her pain was under control as she faded out, waiting for death to take her. The thought felt comforting, but I couldn't help but wonder if this was how she wanted things to end: to be set adrift onto a sea of oblivion, floating in and out of clarity and consciousness, all by herself. It certainly seemed better than dying in a hospital, I thought, or dying in pain. But would this fearless, willful woman have chosen a different path, given the chance? Eventually, I got up and left. Ella died two days later.

My second hospice assignment couldn't have been more different. At a hundred and one years old, Theresa had been living with advanced dementia for ten years. She had cycled through various skilled nursing homes all across Portland until her Medicare ran out. Though her son Steven—a bearlike, unassuming man in his seventies—didn't exactly have the space, he had taken his mother in. Theresa was nonverbal and practically immobile, and she required around-the-clock care. Steven became her full-time caregiver. One day a week, for four hours at a time, I provided respite care for him by looking after his mother so he could leave the house.

When Steven led me into the cramped, poorly lit bedroom he shared with Theresa, the first thing I noticed was the stench of urine coming from the commode. Steven was apologetic, hurrying to empty the bowl into the toilet. I could tell he had tried to straighten up the place before my arrival—a mop sat dripping in the bathroom; the kitchen dishes crowded into a rack. He was trying his best. Theresa lay curled up, her head elevated by a stack of pillows, thin strands of gray hair draped across her white face. She was sleeping. Steven said that his mother was usually active at night and slept during the day. He told me not to step too close; she was prone to biting and lashing out. Once, she had slapped a doctor who tried to examine her.

Steven explained what he wanted me to do while he ran errands and volunteered at the food pantry of his church: sit in the living room, with the bedroom door ajar, and pop in every so often to check on his mother. He shuffled into the kitchen to mix up two bottles of vanilla and chocolate Ensure, which he poured into a plastic mug. Steven stabbed a straw through the lid and stepped back into the bedroom.

"Mom, time for your morning coffee." He raised his voice, trying to sound upbeat but sounding pained instead. "Your morning coffee, Mom!" In a daze, Theresa half opened one eye, a wild stare in her look. Steven pinned the mug into the crease of her left elbow close to her chin so that her mouth could clasp the straw. Theresa took one sip of her shake and dozed off again, the straw burrowing a dent into her cheek.

My time at Steven's house came and went without incident, but it left me profoundly unsettled. Every once in a while, I would hear a deep moaning from the bedroom and would go in to check on Theresa. But she never fully awoke. It pains me to admit that I was glad for it, because I was afraid what would happen if she did. In my mind, Theresa had been reduced to a distant shadow of a person. What was it that made life livable for her? Was it livable? When had she passed the threshold of interceding on her own behalf? And what would her options for choosing a different course have been anyway?

I never found out what happened to Theresa. I had to move back East and was replaced by a new volunteer. But it didn't take much to imagine that Theresa's future wouldn't look so different from her present. She could have kept going like this, potentially for years.

I mention these two hospice assignments not because they are typical ways of dying in America—they are not. Today, 60 percent of Americans die in hospitals, frequently in intensive care units, with very little say about anything.[1] I mention them because at the time I met Ella and Theresa, I was immersed in my research on assisted dying, and I had seen what it can look like to determine the manner and timing of your own death. Like Ella and Theresa, the patients I had come to know suffered from a life-limiting illness. Having run out of treatment options, they had enrolled in hospice. But unlike Ella and Theresa, they were looking for more than hospice could give them. In the midst of seeing their body and sense of self slip away, they sought to maintain some semblance of control.

I am not saying that Ella and Theresa should have had an assisted death. Ella wasn't in a place to discuss her mortality and seemed generally fine with the way things were going. And Theresa would have never been able to qualify for Oregon's assisted dying law, which excludes patients who have lost mental acuity. But their situations caused me to wonder what would have happened if Ella and Theresa hadn't wanted to run out the clock on hospice. Seeing the contrast between their experiences and those of the patients I had met gave me a sharper sense of what an assisted death offers to those for whom hospice doesn't hold all the answers.

Hospice and palliative care have no doubt transformed how we think about and manage the process of dying. Palliative care is an umbrella term for specialized, noncurative medical care that focuses on relieving a seriously ill patient's symptoms through comfort care—symptoms from their disease as well as its treatment. Palliative care specialists begin working with patients in a hospital setting at any stage of their illness, often alongside curative treatment. Once a patient stops treatment and is faced with a finite life expectancy, hospice takes over. As a form of palliative medicine, hospice uses palliative care techniques to reduce suffering at the end of life.

Hospice and palliative care have been at the forefront of a critical paradigm shift away from unnecessary—and often harmful—life-extending measures toward accepting and easing the process of dying. Since the 1970s, they have emerged as an antidote to the excesses of heroic medicine—our growing ability to prolong life through technological intervention, the "more is better" approach of modern medicine. Extraordinary treatments like the mechanical ventilator, developed initially to keep patients alive during intensive surgeries and long reserved for such extreme situations, have become routine interventions today. In *The Art of Dying Well*, Katy Butler shows how hard it can be to step off what she calls "the conveyor belt of fast medicine," which shuttles patients along an assembly line of progressively invasive medical procedures.[2] Mobilizing high-tech medical care at the end of life may give someone a few more days and weeks, but it can also needlessly draw out their suffering.

In America, hospice typically involves in-home services rather than the move to a special facility. As I was told during my training, "hospice is a philosophy rather than a building." To qualify for hospice under Medicare, patients must have a life expectancy of six months or less. They must have stopped any disease-directed treatment that goes beyond symptom control, such as chemotherapy or dialysis. Hospice prioritizes a patient's quality of life over the number of days they have left, offering psychological, physical, emotional, and spiritual support to those who are dying and to their families. The hospice teams I met during my research put the whole patient at the center of their care. They typically included physicians, nurses, social workers, physical therapists, and spiritual advisers. For most patients, enrollment in hospice is short—at the hospice organization where I worked, the average stay was twenty days.

Hospice providers are in a tricky position when it comes to assisted dying. The founding principle of hospice is to neither extend life nor hasten death. And hastening death is exactly what assisted dying laws enable patients to do. Until recently, physicians and volunteers who participated in Oregon's Death with Dignity law referred to an assisted death as a "hastening." They would say, "we're going to a hastening" or "Sally is hastening." The concept points to the idea of expediting an unavoidable fate—dictated by a patient's terminal prognosis—rather than the active cessation of a life that would otherwise continue.

Initially, use of the term "hastening" didn't make it easier for hospice to get on board with the idea of assisted dying. But it wasn't just the term. Linda Downey, former executive director of Willamette Valley Hospice in Salem, explained the challenges hospices faced when assisted dying first became legal in Oregon.

"Patients are reluctant to come on hospice in the first place, usually because it means acknowledging that they're dying," said Downey. "If patients felt that hospice was actively engaged in helping people die, they would be even more reluctant to come on hospice. So we were trying to be very careful."

Palliative care and hospice physicians who oppose assisted dying argue that palliative medicine already offers symptom relief to dying patients—without, however, speeding up their death. Keri Brenner, a palliative care physician and psychiatrist at Stanford, says that palliative care is fully capable of mitigating pain and depression at the end of life.

"We already know there's a better way to die," Brenner testified during a public hearing on a proposed assisted dying bill in Boston in 2017. "More robust and widespread palliative care and hospice are the solution. We cultivate care that actually aligns with patient choices and family values."

As a whole, the palliative care community remains divided on the issue of assisted dying.[3] Many clinicians share Brenner's sense that palliative care can address most suffering, and they worry how their involvement in assisting people to die might be construed.[4] Many are sensitive to a generalized public skepticism toward palliative care based on a popular conflation of palliative care with hospice—patients sometimes interpret their physician's suggestion to start palliative care as an attempt to get them to cease treatment and transition to end-of-life care.[5] Some palliative care physicians fear that their involvement in assisted deaths might worsen these suspicions. Others are a bit humbler about the ability of palliative medicine and hospice to treat all suffering and have welcomed the addition of assisted dying to their toolkit.[6]

According to the law, hospice providers aren't obligated to participate in an assisted death, but they are still in charge of patients who seek out that option. Hospice is responsible for accompanying patients until the time of death and beyond. Since the early days of the Oregon law, many hospice organizations have adopted a position of "studied neutrality" toward assisted dying. They recognized that assisted dying is an end-of-life option that is here to stay, and they didn't want to abandon patients intent on pursuing it. Today, many hospice providers in Oregon try to answer patients' questions about assisted dying and provide them with resources to explore this option on their own. But—by their own policy—they typically can't be present when the patient ingests the lethal medication. However, hospice nurses may wait in an adjacent room and join the family after the death to help with postmortem arrangements.

A small number of hospices support a patient through the process of an assisted death more directly. Kaiser Permanente refers their hospice patients to a patient coordinator inside the Kaiser health system who helps them navigate the path toward an assisted death, often in close cooperation with End of Life Choices Oregon, the volunteer organization that helps patients and families navigate an assisted death. By contrast, most Catholic hospices maintain a strict policy against assisted dying and decline to be involved in any capacity. One of the largest healthcare providers in Oregon is Providence, a Catholic health system that runs several hospitals and hospice services in the state. Providence staff are officially barred from participating in the law, and they may stonewall a dying patient's request to pursue an assisted death. Their refusal to support the practice has led to some significant delays for patients looking to use the law, especially at a moment when timing is of the essence.

Since Oregon passed its Death with Dignity Act in 1997, hospice use in the state has seen significant increases. By 2013, hospice participation among Medicare patients had gone up to 40 percent in Oregon, compared to fewer than 20 percent nationally.[7] That's not an accident. Health systems and state health officials wanted to ensure that assisted dying wasn't going to become a substitute for comprehensive end-of-life care, so they have invested major resources into hospice infrastructure. Nick Gideonse, associate professor of family medicine at Oregon's Health and Science University, says that the expansion of hospice services in Oregon has been a significant collateral benefit of having an assisted dying law on the books.

"I think it was a wonderful effect of the law that we began to have a nice and important competition with hospice and palliative care about best meeting a patient's needs," Gideonse explained. "All the evidence is pretty clear that Oregon's law enhanced all those aspects of care."

In fact, participation in hospice and selecting an assisted death aren't opposing choices. In 2020, close to 95 percent of those who used Oregon's assisted dying law did so as part of a hospice program—theirs was not an either/or decision.[8] If we think of assisted dying not as an alternative but as a complement to hospice, it becomes clear that an assisted death affords dying patients something that a conventional death on hospice does not.

As people approach the end of their life, it can be difficult for them to retain a say over how things should unfold, even if they manage to stay out of a hospital. All too rapidly, lives unravel, events take on a course and logic of their own, and those who are dying may find themselves in a situation they would have never chosen for themselves. Though hospice may take away pain and anxiety and help someone come to terms with the fact that they are dying, hospice deaths don't always succeed in preserving someone's personal sense of autonomy and dignity. And they can be difficult for family members tasked with caring for the dying.

Andrew's wife, Susan, was sixty-two years old when she received a terminal diagnosis of metastatic pancreatic cancer in April 2011. Within a few short months, she was confined to her bed in their North Portland home and came to depend on twenty-four-hour care by her husband, sisters, sons, and the occasional hospice nurse. To this day, Andrew is haunted by the memory of helplessness that marked Susan's dying process. Managing her medications and unpredictable symptoms left the family overwhelmed, even with hospice on standby. Andrew constantly had to strike a bargain between getting a handle on Susan's pain and her desire for mental clarity.

"People don't know what they are in for with hospice," Andrew told me as we sat under the imposing tree of heaven in his backyard. "Near the end, our hospice nurse told me that morphine was our 'best friend,' but I wasn't sure whether I was doing the right thing. I was managing the body of a helpless, dying person who had relinquished all her power to me. I had become an instrument of her will without all of the tools."

Within four months, Susan could no longer make any decisions about the end of her life. Bearing the brunt of the responsibility for her care, Andrew felt inadequate and in over his head. "Hospice connotes a type of beneficence that doesn't always play out, through no fault of their own," he said, his eyes tracing the contours of the leaves overhead. "You can easily lose the thread."

Hospice philosophy recognizes that a terminal diagnosis brings not only physical pain but also social, emotional, and spiritual pain. Dame Cicely Saunders, founder of the first modern hospice in London in 1967, coined the term "total pain" to describe this idea, noting that existential suffering can be just as agonizing as physical pain.

For patients who pursue an assisted death, existential suffering usually overshadows all other concerns, even worries about physical pain. Losing a sense of who and why you are in the world can become a pain so searing, it feels just like an open wound. When dying patients no longer see purpose and meaning in staying alive—when they have only miserable days ahead of them—the prospect of living can feel more daunting than the act of dying.

Physicians who prescribe life-ending medication believe that there are certain kinds of suffering—loss of dignity, loss of bodily control, loss of a sense of self—that are difficult, if not impossible, to allay. Charles Blanke, an oncologist at the Oregon Health and Science University, is convinced that these are the exact situations that hospice cannot palliate. In 2018, he wrote 14 percent of all prescriptions for assisted dying in Oregon, the most of any physician that year.

"I agree that a patient shouldn't take their own life because of inadequate pain control," Blanke told me. "But I've also seen people who have literally no quality of life—an ill patient who can't see friends, can't watch TV, can't read, just lies in bed staring at the ceiling all night, all day. They have nothing to look forward to, and they would prefer not to be alive. I can't think of any way that we can make that concern better. That's suffering. Absolutely."

I knew what Blanke meant. In the course of my research, I had met patients who used to devour a book a day and who could no longer read or even watch TV because their eyes were unable to focus on an image. Patients whose swollen brains made them unable to follow a single conversation. Patients like Joe who spent their days lying frozen in a recliner. They all said their quality of life was zero.

During the final weeks of Susan's life leading up to her death in July, Andrew's wife was no longer the person he remembered.

"Susan's personhood had exhausted itself," he recalled, brushing tears from his cheeks. "And she wasn't able to escape, even within the scope of hospice, the point when life had gone on beyond anything she would have liked. Witnessing an expired person remain in life, strung out on drugs, without physical capacity to digest anything or communicate, it broke my heart. I still know that Susan died in a suffering moment."

Even with the best hospice team and the sheer zeal of Andrew's and her family's care, Susan had a difficult dying process that left Andrew feeling disempowered. Nine years after her death, he still mourns the loss of agency he and his wife experienced at the end of her life.

———————————

Most people who seek an assisted death don't worry about uncontrolled physical pain, but there are those that do. Even inside an advanced medical system, some patients suffer from symptoms that don't respond to the tools of modern medicine: patients whose physical agonies at the end of their life are so relentless, no amount of morphine will touch their pain; patients who vomit feces; patients who are no longer able to digest food and who throw up constantly; patients with neurological pain so blinding, they can't get any relief.

For those extreme situations, hospice does have a way to respond, but it's not very well known or advertised: palliative sedation. Palliative sedation involves sedating a hospice patient who is experiencing unremitting symptoms and whose suffering can't be relieved through any means other than putting them into a coma or on the brink of a coma. With the consent of the patient, a physician administers high doses of narcotics to get on top of their pain.

"You bring them right to the level of comfort through step-by-step sedation," the medical director of a Portland hospice explained. "And sometimes that means unconsciousness."

Sedation to unconsciousness—also known as total sedation—is a measure of last resort usually performed between one to ten days prior to someone's projected time of death. Because food and water are withdrawn at the same time, the patient eventually succumbs to their illness or dies from dehydration.

Unlike assisted dying, palliative sedation became an accepted medical practice without undergoing much public dispute or even scrutiny.[9] Currently, palliative sedation is governed by a standard of care, which means that physicians have come up with their own guidelines rather than having to follow any legal statutes. In fact, it is common practice even in Catholic hospices. That's because palliative sedation makes use of the legal doctrine of "double effect": an action with potentially adverse side effects becomes permissible in pursuit of a greater good. During palliative sedation, the physician's primary goal is to relieve pain, *not* to deliberately cause a patient's death. But if the patient dies in the process of being sedated—which they nearly always do—that's an accepted outcome.[10]

One issue with palliative sedation is that it renders someone unconscious for up to a week before they die, usually inside a clinical institution, while the family holds an unending vigil. For some patients and their loved ones, that doesn't sound like a good option. And besides, palliative sedation is reserved for extraordinary cases of uncontrolled pain, including seizures, vomiting, breathlessness, and bowel obstruction, and most patients with a terminal diagnosis don't fall into that category.

The minute he enrolled in hospice, Joe asked his hospice physician about the possibility of palliative sedation. He was told he didn't qualify—his sporadic air hunger and feeling of drowning weren't viewed as extreme.

"Usually you have to have intractable pain, like from cancer," his partner, Anna, explained. "Hospice doctors must have tried everything they can, and then they will go with palliative sedation, and it would be inpatient. Joe didn't want to be an inpatient, even if he qualified. It wasn't a choice that he would consider."

Joe would have to find a way to end his suffering outside the framework of hospice.

PART II
Navigating Obstacles

CHAPTER 3

Restrictive Laws

When a committee of lawyers, physicians, and activists sat down to craft Oregon's Death with Dignity Act in 1993, they knew they had their work cut out for them. Similar ballot initiatives had recently failed in California and Washington State, and it had been nearly a century since the first bills to ease the dying process for very sick patients had surfaced in state legislatures—with nothing to show. In 1906, legislators in Iowa and Ohio had proposed the "chloroform bills," which envisioned the use of chloroform on fatally ill or injured patients to induce their death. Their terms were so flawed that they never materialized. Other legislative proposals—introduced in Nebraska in 1937, Florida in 1967, and Idaho in 1969—met similar fates.

One sticking point long prevented right-to-die legislation from gaining a foothold in America. So far, all proposals for medical assistance in dying had included a stipulation for euthanasia—the act of a physician ending a patient's life with a lethal injection. The 1991 ballot initiative in Washington State, for example, would have allowed a physician to administer the lethal drugs if the patient could not take them. The measure failed 46 to 54 percent. There was something unpalatable to voters about doctors actively terminating the lives of their patients, even upon request.

Voters weren't the only ones to struggle with the concept. Peter Goodwin, a family physician from Portland, was one of eight members of the Oregon Right to Die committee tasked with drafting the Oregon statute. At the time, Goodwin was still doing house calls, and he had seen the difference between a patient dying at home surrounded by family versus a hospital death—where the patient and family were all too often left without a clear road map. Goodwin noticed that his profession had a difficult time facing the idea of a patient dying. And because he had seen what dying could look like, he wanted patients to have more control over their death.

Goodwin recalled the heated deliberations he and the committee had around the question of euthanasia. "I was insistent that the patient have control, that the patient must take the medication. And that euthanasia, by the doctor injecting the patient, was out."[1]

Goodwin picked up the phone and called thirty family doctors to poll them about their stance on the issue.

"About half of them said 'Yes, under certain circumstances, I could help a dying patient die. But euthanasia? No way.' Not one of them could consider it. Nor could I. I couldn't consider actually causing the death of a patient. I wanted the patient to have that option."

Derek Humphry, also a member of the committee, fought hard to retain a provision for euthanasia. A British-born journalist, Humphry had risen to prominence in 1975 when he helped his wife, Jean, die at their home in England. Jean had been diagnosed with terminal breast cancer four years prior, and she was fearful of dying a painful death. At her request, Humphry laced a cup of coffee with Seconal and codeine and put it on her side table. They kissed goodbye, and Jean picked up the cup and drank it down. Within the hour, she was gone. Humphry's account of her death, *Jean's Way*, became a bestseller in the UK and was translated into eight languages.

Humphry's second marriage took him to California, where he and his new wife, Ann Wickett, founded the Hemlock Society in 1980. Named after the poisonous plant that looks like a wild carrot, the Hemlock Society soon became one of the most renowned right-to-die advocacy organizations in America. Its aim was twofold: to offer its members straightforward information about how to die when their time had come and to get assisted dying legislation passed across the country. Ten years later, Humphry authored *Final Exit*, a practical guide for terminally ill patients on how to end their own lives. Its success was instantaneous: in August 1991, the book lunged to the top of the *New York Times* bestseller list.

When I pulled up to Humphry's secluded home in the Oregon woods, he ushered me into the drafty barn that doubled as his office. Stacks of papers and books were piled ceiling high and the walls covered with faded, framed newspaper clippings of Humphry's professional triumphs. He wore a heavy wool, crimson sweater and steel-gray slacks, his forehead framed by a black visor. At eighty-seven years old,

Humphry was unapologetically eccentric, and he was prone to long digressions. But he remembered the committee's discussions as if they happened yesterday.

"I said we must leave lethal injection in the statute because some people can't swallow," Humphry recalled. "And Peter Goodwin argued that doctors didn't like injecting; they find it repugnant. If we take that out and just have prescriptions, he said, then we will pass. But for me, it's a split ethical point whether I hand you a bottle of pentobarbital or I inject you because you asked me to. Ethically, I think it's exactly the same."

In the end, the committee sided with Goodwin: the Oregon statute would not allow for euthanasia. Under the proposed law, patients would have to ingest the lethal dose themselves.

Anticipating strong opposition to the proposed law—and in the spirit that something is better than nothing—the committee peppered the statute with a long list of restrictions and safeguards. Against Humphry's suggestion to keep the time frame open-ended, the statute specified a condition for terminality: to be eligible for the law, a patient would have to have a terminal disease that put them within six months of the end of their life, as certified by two physicians.

The attending (or "prescribing") physician would carry the burden of responsibility of qualifying a patient for the law: they would determine whether a patient meets the eligibility requirements, inform the patient of feasible alternatives and their right to rescind their request, ensure that the patient is making an informed decision, put together the documentation, and write the prescription and send it to a pharmacy.

The consulting physician would independently examine the patient and their medical records and confirm the attending physician's diagnosis.

In addition to being an Oregon resident and over the age of eighteen, a patient would have to demonstrate medical decision-making capacity to qualify for an assisted death (or be referred to a mental health expert for further scrutiny). Physicians and pharmacists could decline to participate in the law, with no obligation to refer the patient to a different provider. The statute also introduced a fifteen-day waiting period between a patient's first and second oral request, intended as a period of reflection or "cooling off." At some point after their first oral request, a patient would have to file a written request signed by two witnesses. It is only forty-eight hours after receiving the written request that the attending physician could issue a prescription for life-ending medication (but not before the fifteen-day waiting period had concluded).[2]

It worked. In 1994, Oregonians narrowly approved the Death with Dignity Act at the ballot box. But because the margin was razor thin (51 percent in favor and 49 percent opposed), opponents filed a legal injunction that prevented the statute from being enacted. During the stay, in 1997, the U.S. Supreme Court ruled that terminally ill patients do not have a constitutionally protected right to medical assistance in dying—individual states would have to create their *own* assisted dying laws. Later that year, on October 27, 1997, the Ninth Circuit Court of Appeals lifted the injunction on the original act.

The opposition immediately attempted to repeal the original statute. During a special election that November, voters were asked to revoke the measure once and for all. They didn't. Oregonians came out in strong favor of the act by a 20 percent margin. For the first time in American history, terminally ill patients had a legal way to end their own lives.

It took another eleven years for a second state to follow suit. At the end of a contentious campaign, voters in Washington State affirmed their support for their own Death with Dignity Act in 2008, which was closely modeled after Oregon's law. Since then, nearly every state that has legalized medical assistance in dying has either followed the Oregon model or, in the case of Hawaii, added more constraints to it.[3]

More than twenty years into the legalization of assisted dying in America, these laws remain the most restrictive in the world.[4] Intended to reduce unnecessary suffering, they sometimes have the opposite effect. Every year, hundreds of eligible patients who apply for an assisted death are so close to the end of their life, they die during the mandated waiting period that kicks in after their first oral request. Many wade through the dense bureaucracy of these laws while their energy and health are fast declining. Patients with open-ended degenerative diseases, like Parkinson's or ALS, cannot qualify unless they are within imminent reach of their death. And those at risk of losing their ability to self-administer the lethal medication worry constantly that they might miss the precious window when they are able to take the drugs.

The Oregon statute and other statutes that came after it use verbs like "ingest" or "take" to describe the process of self-administration. Most physicians have interpreted this language to allow for any method that involves a person's digestive system—including through a feeding tube or a rectal catheter—provided that the patient self-administers the medication.

George Eighmey, former executive director of Compassion in Dying of Oregon, knows that the rule around self-administration is one of the most onerous parts of the law. But he also believes it is one of the most important.

"Nobody can pour it down your throat; nobody can inject you; nobody can pour it down your feeding tube," he said in an interview with historian Richard Côté. "You must be physically able to end your life without an assistant. That means many people who meet all the other qualifications fall through the gap because they are too sick to take the medicine."[5]

Eighmey is the first to point out the paradox of his position: terminally ill patients, the very people for whom the law is intended, cannot use it if they are too sick. But Eighmey still thinks it's worth it to have the law. Trained as a lawyer, Eighmey became an activist for the right-to-die movement during the height of the HIV/AIDS epidemic in the 1980s, which was ravaging the lives of young gay men. He witnessed many of them commit suicide because they had no legal means of ending their lives to escape a ghastly death. Eighmey spent years lobbying lawmakers to draft legislation that would give dying patients a better way out.

When we talked, Eighmey said that the requirement for self-administration guarantees that a patient acts of their own accord. The involvement of another person could lead to abuse and into pressuring a patient into a death they did not want or for which they weren't ready. "We wanted to make sure that the vulnerable weren't in any way coerced," Eighmey explained. "So we came up with the term 'self-determination, self-administration,' and it caught on."

Some prescribing physicians see the value in retaining the current restrictions, even if they know that a patient's timeline is driven forward by the rule for self-administration. Nick Gideonse, associate professor of family medicine at Oregon's Health and Science University, recognizes the importance of maintaining the directive in place.

"It's a final guarantee of voluntariness," said Gideonse. "I'm still comfortable with that being a public good. Occasionally, I've seen people definitely shorten their lives substantially based on that single requirement. And I regret that. But it's a public policy that has preserved a lot of good for a lot of people."

And yet Gideonse acknowledges that the rule could feel ethically arbitrary. "I've provided the prescription, right? I am helping the person die. If you were to ask me to administer the drugs through a push of a syringe, I don't fundamentally feel that changes my position very much at all."

Other physicians are unhappy about these limitations. They point to the experience of other countries with assisted dying laws, which shows that administering the drugs through the bloodstream by a clinician is much faster, safer, and more effective.

"I want a Canadian law," Neil Martin, Ken's physician, told me. "I think it's ridiculous to have our law written such that you have to be able to swallow the medication on your own. So many neurodegenerative diseases work against that. So many cancers work against that. You are discriminating, inadvertently, based on disease process and physical ability. If you're creating a law for truly trying to help patients end their suffering, what difference does it make if the drugs are administered by a physician or self-administered?"

In Canada, which legalized assisted dying in 2016, qualified patients can choose between a self-administered death and a lethal injection by a clinician. So far, their preferences have been unequivocal: between January and October of 2018, more than 99 percent opted for an injection, for which the average time to death is ten minutes.[6] In the Netherlands and in Belgium, injections are also the norm. All three countries, along with Switzerland, Colombia, and Luxembourg, place the emphasis on a patient's current suffering—rather than on their projected life expectancy—to qualify them for the law. That means they allow for more open-ended prognoses and, in some cases, psychological suffering.

Elizabeth Steiner Hayward, a physician and state senator in Oregon, says that assisted dying laws *should* be difficult to access to prevent abuse and false accusations. Steiner Hayward has served as both a prescribing and consulting physician under the law, and she understands the complicated politics around assisted dying.

"There's the letter of the law, the spirit of the law, and then there's who is going to talk about it," she told me. "All of us who are involved with this law are very cautious, because our opponents are looking for any reason to say that we are killing off people with disabilities. We are incredibly careful."

Over the years, the Oregon statute has withstood an onslaught of legal challenges. In 2006, the U.S. Supreme Court upheld the rights of physicians to prescribe controlled substances under the law after Attorney General John Ashcroft threatened to prosecute them. Despite several proposed amendments to the law, the original statute has changed very little, with one exception. In 2019, Oregon legislators voted to expedite the fifteen-day waiting period for patients judged by their attending physician to be *in extremis*—at the point of death. If the physician thinks that a patient has less than two days to live, the standard forty-eight-hour wait between a patient's written request and the writing of their prescription can also be waived.

Even though assisted dying laws in America are relatively restrictive, most opponents of the practice believe they are much too permissive. The potential for coercion and abuse, they say, lurks everywhere. Critics argue that assisted dying laws allow physicians to give up on their patients prematurely, pressure the elderly and people with disabilities to end their lives, and enable families to murder a loved one with impunity.

"The entire thing is under a shroud of secrecy," said Bill Toffler, a family physician at the Oregon Health and Science University and an outspoken opponent of medical assistance in dying. "It's the perfect murder. Once you have the overdose, there's nobody witnessing to see what happens with it."

Toffler is the director of Physicians for Compassionate Care, a nonprofit that campaigns against assisted dying laws. He says he doesn't have any hope that the Oregon law would be repealed in his lifetime, but he hopes to keep it from spreading. For Toffler, there are no safeguards in the world that could make him change his mind; his opposition is one of principle.

None of the law's opponents I spoke with said there could ever be enough protections for them to morally condone medical assistance in dying. Lois Anderson, executive director of Oregon Right to Life, certainly doesn't think there could be. She believes that no human life should end prematurely—no matter the circumstances. Like Toffler, Anderson has no hope of reversing the law ("If I were dreaming big, sure!"), but she is trying to limit its damage by educating people on the intrinsic value of life.

"There is so much complexity to the human experience that I don't think you can create safeguards that can be effective in every single situation," she said when we sat down in her office. The office building was so inconspicuous, I had driven past it twice. In a state that goes reliably liberal every election year, her organization was trying to keep a low public profile. "All life should be protected. At some point, you're going to end up with a dead person that shouldn't have died or that didn't want to die."

Kenneth Stevens is of a similar mind. A former chair of radiation oncology at the Oregon Health and Science University, Stevens cofounded Physicians for Compassionate Care with Toffler. Stevens felt proud to have helped keep the Oregon law from expanding to other states for over ten years. And he scoffed at the question of protections.

"My medical conscience says I cannot purposely harm my patient," Stevens told me. "My patients should be in a safe haven when they're receiving care from their doctor."

But it wasn't just Stevens's medical conscience that drove his opposition. It was also his religious conscience. Stevens identifies as Mormon, and the Mormon Church strictly opposes assisted dying. His colleague Bill Toffler shares his religiously grounded opposition to the law. Toffler is a devout Catholic—so devout, he doesn't prescribe birth control pills to his female patients. But Toffler was careful about using religious language to explain why he is against the law. "If you say life is sacred, our culture will say that you're a religious nut," Toffler told me. "I do believe life is sacred, but I also believe it's inherently valuable."

Critics of assisted dying tend to downplay the religious aspects of their opposition to avoid alienating nonbelievers. During one public hearing on a proposed assisted dying bill in Massachusetts, I overheard two ministers who testified for the opposition say they would never dare show up in a clerical collar, while proponents were free to do so.

Canadian anthropologist Ari Gandsman explains why opponents are hesitant to showcase their religious convictions publicly. "Activists believe that if the right-to-die debate is reduced to the question of one side imposing religious beliefs on others in a secular society, they will lose," he notes.[7] Instead of making absolute moral claims, opponents have taken up a new rhetoric of risk and uncertainty, intended to sow doubt about the true purpose behind assisted dying laws.

The "slippery slope" argument is a centerpiece of this strategy. Many opponents argue that once you open the door to an assisted death, even narrowly at first, it will eventually swing wide open and cause irreparable societal harm. Today, people who are terminally ill are using the law; tomorrow, it will be everyone who is elderly, disabled, or poor. Assisted dying may start out as voluntary, but it will soon lead to people requesting to die due to rising societal, familial, and financial pressures.

John Kelly, a disability rights advocate from Boston, argues that assisted dying laws already embody a deadly form of discrimination against people with disabilities. He is the New England regional director of Not Dead Yet, a nonprofit that lobbies against assisted dying legislation. During an October 2017 visit to one of my college classes, Kelly told students that medical assistance in dying implicitly devalues the lives of people with disabilities, who must live daily with the same limitations terminally ill patients try to escape by seeking an assisted death. Kelly said that the top reasons assisted dying patients give for wanting to die are the "quintessential definition of what it means to be disabled." Rather than continuing to receive assistance to live, Kelly claimed, people with disabilities would soon be folded into assisted dying laws and subtly encouraged to end their lives.

Despite allegations of coercion and abuse, the official state record in Oregon shows no instances of malfeasance. As a prescribing physician, Gideonse thinks it would be incredibly difficult to force the law on someone, given the many hurdles a patient must clear to qualify.

"You would think some grieving family members would have come forward if they felt that their grandmother never would have left them if she wasn't coerced. It just hasn't happened. How do you make someone drink something they don't want to drink? It's incredibly bitter—you can't just sneak it in."

Even so, Oregon's Death with Dignity Act contains several gaps and gray areas, and it leaves some issues unaddressed. Though the law requires a patient to self-administer the lethal dose, the statute is silent on how exactly an assisted death ought to proceed once a patient has obtained the prescription.

"The statute only addresses what happens up to the point the prescription is written," Katrina Hedberg, state epidemiologist at the Oregon Health Authority, told me when we spoke in 2018. The Oregon Health Authority is the central state body that collects all statistics on assisted dying and ensures that physicians and patients follow the letter of the law. Physicians who sign off on an assisted death are required to document each case and submit the paperwork to the agency. Hedberg oversaw the law's reporting system from 1997 to 2019.

"The statute does not address anything that needs to happen after the prescription is written. You can get the prescription if you meet the qualifications at the time, but it doesn't say anything about what might happen if people lose cognitive abilities some months later. None of this is addressed in the statute."

The law has no mechanism for reassessing a patient after the prescription is issued. Someone could receive the prescription and later become ineligible based on a loss of bodily or mental function. In practice, patients who lose competence end up not using the medication.

Once they can no longer swallow or push the drugs through a feeding tube, they understand that it's too late. And patients who become mentally incompetent aren't in a place to ask their caregiver for the medication, much less answer the three standard questions a physician (if one is present) would ask them before preparing the lethal dose: Whose decision is this? What will happen if you take this medicine? Do you want to change your mind? If a patient doesn't respond satisfactorily, or if the physician picks up on any hesitation in their voice, they postpone or annul the death.

If a physician isn't present, volunteers often serve as the final gatekeepers for an assisted death. They may be the ones responsible for putting on the brakes, even if a patient has already qualified for the law and obtained the medication. Volunteers follow their own protocol that says a patient must verbalize what they are about to do and must be in their right mind before proceeding. Above all, volunteers want to ensure that someone doesn't feel pressured to move ahead—even after calling their loved ones together.

A handful of times, Derianna, the volunteer who attended Ken's death, had to postpone an assisted death because a patient was unable to fully articulate what would happen if they drank the lethal cocktail. One time, a patient told her that the life-ending drugs would make him feel a lot better tomorrow. *Wrong answer*, Derianna thought, her heart sinking. She suspected that his pain medications had temporarily fogged his mind, and she told the family that today was not the day. She offered to reschedule until a time when he could be taken off the medications for a few hours to clear his thoughts.

The law doesn't insist on this safeguard, because a patient can carry out an assisted death without the attendance of a volunteer or physician.[8] Many people, however, do have help. In 2019, 57 percent of all assisted deaths in Oregon were attended by a physician, another healthcare provider, or a volunteer. Between 1998 and the end of 2018, a physician or healthcare provider accompanied roughly 40 percent of all assisted deaths in the state—and volunteers aren't included in that statistic. Until 2019, the Oregon Health Authority didn't collect any data on nonmedical providers present at an assisted death, despite the critical role they play.

Assisted dying laws also don't specify what should happen to unused medications. To find answers, people must look to sources outside the statutes. Pharmacies recommend treating life-ending medications like any other controlled substance and returning unused doses to a take-back program. Alternatively, loved ones can take the medications out of their original containers, mix them with an undesirable substance—like wet coffee grounds or kitty litter—and place them into a sealed bag in the trash. That way, the medications won't enter the water supply.

Finally, it is unclear what should happen if a patient who ingested the life-ending drugs regains consciousness after falling into a coma. Could they receive additional sedatives to keep them unconscious until they die? Who would administer them? Who is responsible for a patient who awakens? And would the patient have to restart the application process, or could they simply receive a new set of drugs?[9]

Even if these gaps didn't exist, it's never enough to simply have a law—you need people to help implement it. Assisted dying laws provide a blueprint of conditions that patients and practitioners must meet, but they don't outline concrete procedures or provide state resources for going about an assisted death.

Since the early days of the law, much of this work has fallen on volunteer organizations. In the Pacific Northwest, the volunteer model has persisted as the primary source of support for patients and families seeking an assisted death. Initially, volunteers were part of Compassion in Dying, an advocacy group that merged with the Hemlock Society to become Compassion and Choices in 2005. Increasingly focused on winning legal battles across the country, Compassion and Choices gradually moved away from letting volunteers attend the deaths of their clients for fear of legal repercussions.

In 2015, most of their volunteers in Washington State spun off and founded their own nonprofit, End of Life Washington. Volunteers felt frustrated by the growing restrictions placed on the most important aspect of their work: their personal interactions with patients and families. In 2017, Compassion and Choices volunteers in Oregon arrived at the same conclusion and founded End of Life Choices Oregon. Today, the organization supports an estimated 90 percent of all patients who pursue an assisted death under Oregon's law. Both organizations have built an expansive state-wide network of trained volunteers who help patients and their families manage the path toward an assisted death, acting in an advisory, nonmedical capacity. Perhaps most importantly, volunteers have recruited a group of physicians, many retired and working pro bono, who are willing to examine patients and evaluate their request for an assisted death.

It is precisely the involvement of physicians and the medical system that lends medically assisted deaths a significant measure of social and moral legitimacy—a quality absent in cases where terminally ill people use "do-it-yourself" methods outside the law to end their own lives. The participation of medical professionals also improves the chances for a successful outcome, taking the guess work out of a potentially daunting project. Despite the fact that assisted dying laws are difficult to use, many people prefer staying inside the law and having a medically and legally sanctioned death.

Nevertheless, the mere fact that assisted dying is now legal in many states doesn't mean that anyone can access these laws or that an assisted death can happen out in the open. Twenty-plus years into the legalization of assisted dying in America, the cultural stigma around these laws remains potent.

CHAPTER 4

Invisible Death

In today's America, someone may go their entire life without ever seeing a dead body or witnessing a death. Most people die in nursing homes and hospitals, and funeral professionals handle human remains, keeping death at a safe distance. This removal of the living from the dying process, and from death itself, has intensified a much broader cultural discomfort with our mortality. Not many people feel comfortable talking openly about death. As a result, death has become almost invisible—sequestered in hospitals and mortuaries, outsourced to professionals, muzzled in everyday conversation. Caitlin Doughty, the mortician and author, calls this phenomenon "death dystopia"—the silence, denial, and repression that shroud American society's contemporary engagement with death.[1]

It wasn't always this way. Until the end of the nineteenth century, Americans were far more familiar with many aspects of death because most people died at home, and families took care of their own dead. But it's not just that people usually don't see death up close anymore. Today, the end of life has become so medicalized that death is frequently seen as a failure rather than an expected stage of life. In the face of societal pressures toward staying young and fit, and a nearly unshakable trust in the power of medicine, death has come to be seen as an enemy to be defeated.

The surgeon Atul Gawande argues that this narrow view of death has resulted in people dying in institutions, cut off from loved ones and the comforts of home. "I am in a profession that has succeeded because of its ability to fix," he writes. "If your problem is fixable, we know just what to do. But if it's not? The fact that we have had no adequate answers to this question is troubling and has caused callousness, inhumanity, and extraordinary suffering."[2]

That death has become something many Americans suppress is evident elsewhere too. We see it in the cultural fixation on fantasies of immortality. Some are benign—like antiaging creams or stories about immortal vampires—but others are not. The past two decades have witnessed a burst of efforts to bypass age-related decline in search of eternal life. These include attempts to continue to live virtually by downloading a person's brain or becoming a "ghost bot"—a computer-generated simulation of the deceased that can interact with the living. Then there's the growing field of cryonics, the freezing and storing of bodies or body parts in the hope that future scientists will thaw them and bring them back to life.

These fantasies aren't surprising in a culture that has declared death a scandal.

"We act as if [death does] not exist," writes historian Philippe Ariès, "and thus mercilessly force the bereaved to say nothing."[3]

There's nothing inevitable about this view. People across the world respond to human mortality in different ways. In societies where death is a subject of everyday conversation and where people spend time intentionally preparing for the end of their life, there's a far greater acceptance of death. Among a group of people in West Papua, Indonesia, elders spontaneously speak of themselves as being in the process of dying, notes anthropologist Rupert Stasch. "Aged men, if they are awake before dawn, often sing softly about their upcoming deaths," he writes.[4] Among many Buddhists, dying is seen as an intricate art to be studied, and many Buddhists contemplate death and dying as part of their daily meditation practice. In Mexico, the annual Días de los Muertos, Days of the Dead, not only honor the deceased but provide an open, public space for the bereaved to confront their personal loss and grief.[5]

The cultural taboos that prevent a candid engagement with death in America compound the challenges dying patients face today—from physicians who trade in euphemisms and wishful thinking to the cultural imperative to never give up. A pervasive culture of death denial makes the end of life even harder on people who want to control the manner and terms of their own death. Even in states where medical assistance in dying has long been legal, like Oregon and Washington, patients who seek an assisted death find themselves on uncertain moral ground.

Religious objections to assisted dying account for some of this resis-tance. Many opponents of assisted dying laws in America say that it is against God's design to hasten death, insisting that the intentional taking of a human life is always wrong.[6] James Driscoll, executive direc-tor of the Massachusetts Catholic Conference, asked legislators during a 2015 hearing on Beacon Hill to reject a proposed assisted dying bill for that very reason.

"The Catholic Church teaches that life is a gift from God and should be cherished and nurtured until natural death," Driscoll proclaimed, "not predetermined death based on a diagnosis of terminal illness."

Many religiously motivated opponents argue that patients who pursue an assisted death hijack God's power over life and death—they violate the sacredness of life and short-circuit necessary processes of human struggle. In line with Christian ideas that relate suffering to the prospect of redemption, critics view the ordeals dying patients face as critical opportunities for spiritual growth. They say there's virtue in enduring suffering at the end of life instead of taking what they see as "the easy way out."

It is this position that has led most Catholic health systems to maintain strict policies against assisted dying and bar their clinicians from participating in the law. Especially in rural parts of Oregon east of the Cascades and along the coastal corridor—where Catholic health systems often run the only hospital in town—patients routinely strug-gle to find two physicians who will assess their request.

But despite official policies, individual clinicians are sometimes sympathetic to patients' wish for an assisted death, and they try to connect them to the appropriate resources. They may, for example, contact an advocacy organization for assistance on behalf of a patient, stepping off the premises to place the call from their private cell phones. But it depends on the person, and if a patient has a nurse who is firmly opposed to the law, their quest for an assisted death might run into the sand.

There's another reason why an assisted death comes with a vague sense of deviancy: it is often conflated with the idea of suicide. Until just recently, the primary term in the English language for a purposeful, voluntary death was "suicide." People lacked other, more nuanced vocabulary to think about other forms of intentional self-death, and many still find it hard to shake the stigma and sense of transgression that cling to the idea of ending one's own life.

The popular conflation of assisted dying with suicide isn't only an issue of semantics. Language matters. How we talk about something determines how we think about it conceptually. Calling an assisted death a "suicide" has been harmful to patients and families. It has led to patients hiding their desire to use the law for fear of being judged for "suiciding" and family members feeling isolated in the bereavement process. Some families whose loved one underwent an assisted death were told by members of their hospice grief group, "Oh well, your husband suicided." Afraid of being shamed for allowing their loved one to die, some have had to swallow their grief.

Until well into the nineteenth century, suicide was considered a crime in America, punishable with confiscation of the deceased's property and denial of a Christian burial. Long viewed as an affront to God, the state, and society, suicide gradually became decriminalized and moved under the scope of clinical psychology—which classified it as a pathological desire to end one's life, often as a result of a mental disorder, particularly depression. Although suicide is no longer primarily seen as a sin or a crime, it remains heavily stigmatized. As philosopher Ian Hacking writes, "News of a suicide among us has an immediate response: horror."[7]

Critics argue that calling an assisted death anything other than a suicide is euphemistic, aimed only at sanitizing the practice. During a 2015 public hearing on a proposed assisted dying bill at the State House in Boston, opponents made a point of inviting testimonies by those who had lost someone to suicide or who had been active in suicide-prevention organizations. Mary Hoge, an elder law attorney from Medfield, warned legislators: "If you pass this law, you will redefine a tragedy and call it a medical procedure. You will call death just another choice. We all know suicide has been considered a sad consequence of depression, loneliness, fear, and desperation. Suicide of any kind is a result of a mind in turmoil, an act of a person who feels unloved and abandoned. Can we legislate love and accompaniment instead?"

Similar to Hoge, opponents routinely paint patients who pursue what they call "doctor-prescribed suicide" as plagued by undiagnosed depression or social abandonment.[8] By equating an assisted death with suicide, critics tap into the social taboos and moral outrage that continue to beset the act of taking one's life.

In recent years, supporters of assisted dying laws in America have become increasingly invested in drawing a robust line between assisted dying and a suicidal act. The distinctions they invoke go beyond a simple search for legitimacy or an attempt to distance themselves from the societal stigma that still surrounds suicide in America today. Advocates say that an assisted death warrants a conceptual category of its own. As part of the same hearing that featured Hoge, Carl Brownsberger, a physician from Belmont, Massachusetts, got up to speak. He stepped up to the podium and cleared his throat.

"I've devoted my career mainly to suicide prevention, but these patients aren't suicidal," the doctor declared. "They don't want to die—their death is coming down a train track toward them, and it seems like it's true reverence to life to give them some kind of control over the timing and means of their death."

The Massachusetts bill never advanced to the next round, neither in 2015 nor in 2017. But right-to-die activists across the state welcomed the statement released by the American Association of Suicidology (AAS) on October 30, 2017. The statement asserted that "suicide and physician aid-in-dying are conceptually, medically, and legally different phenomena," so placing medically assisted deaths as matters "outside the central focus of the AAS." For activists, the statement represented a hopeful step toward shifting the terms of a public conversation that continues to lump assisted dying together with the terminology and morality of suicide. As Roger Kligler, a physician-patient who unsuccessfully sued Massachusetts for his right to die, told me: "Calling it suicide means that we're not talking about end-of-life issues."

Legally, an assisted death is not registered as a suicide. Assisted dying laws across America have made a clear distinction between assisted dying and a suicidal act. The nation's first statute, Oregon's Death with Dignity Act, specifies that "Actions taken in accordance with [the Act] shall not, for any purpose, constitute suicide, assisted suicide, mercy killing or homicide, under the law." The death certificate of patients who use assisted dying laws must list their underlying condition as the cause of death, making no mention of either assisted dying or suicide.[9]

For Peter Goodwin, one of the architects of the Oregon law, what made assisted dying different from suicide was that an assisted death takes place inside the medical care system, following medical protocol. "These are patients taking some medication, which we have prescribed according to a proposed law. I have always thought of this as a rational response to a medical problem. And it is the most—it is one of the deepest medical problems. Perhaps the deepest medical problem is how to deal rationally with terminally ill patients."[10]

From their inception, assisted dying laws in America were designed to make an assisted death a routine—if rare—medical practice aimed at easing suffering at the end of someone's life. In fact, medical professionals are charged with upholding a distinction between an assisted death and suicide in their clinical work by screening for mental illness, especially depression. Doctors must weed out "suicidal" patients from those whose desire to die springs legitimately from their terminal diagnosis. If a patient shows any signs of mental impairment, they must undergo further scrutiny by a mental health expert.

Psychiatrists Bostwick and Cohen note that it is precisely the participation of medicine and a patient's social network that differentiates assisted deaths from a suicidal act. An assisted death is collaborative and socially sanctioned—not unilateral and covert. "When they acquiesce to requests to facilitate dying, [physicians] are not abetting suicide or committing homicide," the two authors argue. "The distinction between clinical suicide and other types of end-of-life decisions demands a new formulation."[11]

Peter Reagan, the first Oregon physician whose prescription of life-ending medication led to a patient's assisted death in 1998, agrees with this reasoning. He still remembers riding his bike sixty blocks to his patient's house in Southeast Portland to hand deliver her prescription. Reagan said that using the term suicide to talk about assisted dying is misleading.

"There are so many associations bundled with the concept of suicide that don't pertain to assisted dying: clandestine, illegal, traumatic, ugly, shocking, unexpected, lonely, senseless. The word has a lot of unnecessary baggage. But if you're talking to your family and inviting them to your death and taking a medicine in the presence of other people, it's a whole different thing."

Absent a terminal prognosis, patients who seek an assisted death have no independent desire to end their life. And they are not terminating a life that would otherwise continue—at least not for long.

Miriam's life partner of twenty-four years used Oregon's assisted dying law in 2012 after a debilitating struggle with ALS. As Miriam recounted the progression from Eva's diagnosis to her death in their Portland home, she wanted to make sure I understood one thing about Eva.

"Eva had a wonderful life," Miriam told me. "She did *not* want to die. But she knew where this disease was going. This law isn't being misused by someone who wants to commit suicide. There are so many opportunities if you want to commit suicide. You don't need to use the Death with Dignity statute—which is not easy, which is convoluted, which has its bureaucratic checks and balances. You just wouldn't choose to do it this way."

———————

The widespread moral ambivalence and religious opposition toward assisted dying have majorly complicated its implementation. Especially in the early days of the law, patients and families had the dull sense that their participation in Oregon's Death with Dignity Act was somehow illicit. Most physicians refused to participate in the law back then, and almost no pharmacists were willing to fill a prescription for life-ending medication, or they would only do so after hours, when all their regular customers had left. At the time, there was a lot of sneaking around.

When Doreen went through the process of helping to qualify her husband, Michael, for the law in 2005, they had to drive five hours from Medford in southern Oregon to Portland to meet with the only doctor who had agreed to see him. Michael's exposure to Agent Orange during the Vietnam War had caused him to develop throat cancer at age fifty-three. He underwent surgery and radiation to remove his tumor. Surgeons then placed a permanent tracheostomy tube in his throat, which required him to use an electro-larynx, an electronic device he held up to his throat to speak. Two years later, the cancer returned and he risked losing both his voice box and one of his legs if he underwent surgery again. Michael decided he had had enough and initiated his application for an assisted death. Both he and Doreen were surprised by what came next.

"Back then, you had to go to a very specific doctor," Doreen recalled. "We had to go to 'Dr. Jones' at this location. It was very hush-hush."

After securing a second opinion, the doctor signed off on Michael's request. He warned Doreen and Michael not to say anything to the front staff at his office when they came back for the prescription. "Just say you want to see me," he told them.

Three weeks later, Doreen and Michael went back to his office to pick up a prescription for Nembutal—a barbiturate in liquid form that is no longer available as of this writing—and listened carefully as the doctor laid out which pharmacist at which pharmacy would fill it. Doreen called the pharmacist who had more instructions for her.

"I want you to come in on Monday at ten minutes past six," he said. "We close at six o'clock. My staff should be gone by then. Don't come before six."

Even though the majority of Oregonians had voted for the law in 1994 and again in 1997, opponents of assisted dying were vocal and well organized. Physicians and pharmacists were reluctant to showcase their involvement in the law for fear of losing business, alienating their staff and clients, and attracting picketers to their office. They didn't want to take any chances, even if they supported the legislation in principle.

Sometimes a single pharmacist could foil a patient's ability to get the medication. One woman from Philomath who had qualified for the law rode her mobility scooter four miles to the nearest pharmacy—only to be turned away by the Catholic pharmacist who worked the counter that day. She had received a terminal breast cancer diagnosis in her sixties after a lifelong struggle with polio. Once she qualified for assisted dying, she felt strongly about picking up the drugs herself. When the pharmacist refused to dispense the medication that was waiting for her, she scooted home, called her nurse, and went back the next day with a pair of clinicians.

Finding a permissible place to die was another hurdle. Because the law prohibits patients from taking the lethal medication in a public space, they have to find a private one. Most adult foster homes in the Pacific Northwest forbid the practice under their roof, as do many assisted living facilities and nursing homes. Patients are then forced to make alternative arrangements, compelling them into secrecy and sometimes deception.

Derianna once helped a woman die whose adult foster home wouldn't allow an assisted death on their premises. Out of options, her children booked a room at a Holiday Inn Express and told hotel staff they were hosting a party for their mom's ninety-fourth birthday. Her children specified that they wanted a room close to an exit on the first floor. What they didn't tell staff was the reason for their request: to make it easier for the funeral home to retrieve their mother's body on a gurney.

Family members flew in from across the country and Canada, bringing in flowers and cake. Everyone sat in a circle around the woman's bed and reminisced about her life. Derianna said it was pure joy to watch her family nurture her out.

After her death, her daughters walked up to the front desk and told the hotel manager that their mother had unexpectedly passed away.

"The party was just too much for Mom," they told him.

It isn't ill intentions that are driving families and volunteers to act discreetly—it's the knowledge that their participation must remain private to protect those who are using the law and to spare those who want nothing to do with it. Because of the delicacy of their job and the enduring cultural taboos that beleaguer the act of taking one's own life, the work of volunteers often happens in the shadows. They don't walk around advertising what they do. Even so, volunteers know that they must stay strictly inside the confines of the law. During a volunteer training I attended, a senior volunteer empathically reminded the new recruits, "We need to *protect* the law. Don't jump over the law."

Since those early days, a lot has changed. In 2020, 142 physicians across Oregon wrote prescriptions for assisted dying, and a handful of pharmacies now handle all prescriptions for life-ending medications and ship them to their destination.[12] In the last five years, some assisted living facilities and retirement homes have created policies to support residents who want to use the law, and very few assisted deaths happen in motels anymore. But that doesn't mean all moral objections to the law have evaporated.

Even though assisted dying remains tinged with stigma and accessing it can be a challenge, an assisted death embodies many people's ideal of dying well. Historically, ideas of what makes a "good death" have undergone significant shifts. Originally, the word euthanasia—derived from the Greek words *eu* (good or well) and *thanatos* (death)—meant a good death. Between the late Middle Ages and the Enlightenment, a good death wasn't necessarily a painless death; it was a death "blessed with the grace of God."[13] At the time, popular manuals on the art of dying, *ars moriendi*, coached readers on how to act on their deathbed to ensure their salvation. Priests who were called to the bed of the dying used the manuals to help prepare the pious for their death. It was only once physicians replaced clergy at the deathbed in the course of the nineteenth century that the term euthanasia came to signify a painless death. At the end of that century, euthanasia took on the meaning it still has today: the use of lethal medications at the hands of a clinician to bring about a quick, painless death.

Today, most Americans die in hospitals, and many have come to think of a hospital death as the quintessential "bad death"—a protracted and possibly desperate death, amid machines and strangers in a sterile hospital suite. With the growing use of ventilators and devices that replace the beating function of the human heart, medicine now has an unprecedented capacity to prolong life and manipulate death—even after someone has lost all traces of awareness and cognition. Life-extending technologies have not only redefined what it means to die, they have also created a new problem: death itself has become almost unrecognizable.[14]

In the face of medicine's unparalleled ability to stretch the end of someone's life, the wish for a "good death" continues to gain cultural momentum. For the people I met in the course of my work, a good death typically meant an absence of suffering: a peaceful, gentle parting in a familiar and comfortable place, with the chance to say goodbye. If you asked Derianna, a good death is one where everyone who wants to be present has assembled at the dying person's bedside, feels prepared, and has reached a certain level of acceptance.

"They're grieving, they're horribly grieving, but they are so grateful to be there. It's something that everybody is doing together. To watch someone die, in front of you, I think is not as hard as what your mind does if they die away from you. It's a ritual of witnessing."

An assisted death comes very close to these ideals. It allows dying patients to feel in control over their death because of their ability to time and direct the dying process. Knowing when, where, and how they will die also enables patients to plan for a special kind of departure. They get to choose what they want to wear, whom they would like to invite, and what their final moments will be. Some families develop their own rituals to ease a dying patient's passing and facilitate the process of letting go. Many try to realize their own version of a "good death"—a tender, but occasionally festive, home death in front of an intimate audience of loved ones.

Then there's the death itself. An assisted death seldom involves writhing, incontinence, or seizures; it mimics the process of someone dying calmly in their sleep. Even though a person uses medications to accomplish this goal, an assisted death ends up looking very much like a "natural" death—if all goes well.

––––––

The ability to anticipate death with so much precision has also brought changes to the mortuary industry. Deon Strommer, director of First Call Mortuary Services in Portland, says that clients who are planning an assisted death usually have very specific instructions for him. He once took a call from a customer who knew exactly what he wanted. The client told Strommer, "I'm going to take the medicine by noon. They say I will be dead by three. If you come by at six, that would be a good time. My family will have had enough time."

Strommer, an old-timey gentleman with broad features and a resounding laugh, has been in the mortuary business for decades. A former cattle rancher from central Oregon, he has kept up with the times. Two weeks before my visit, he had bought the first unit for alkaline hydrolysis in Oregon, a new way of disposing of human remains that uses heat, water, and potash inside a steel capsule. His mortuary was right across from Providence Hospital in Northeast Portland, separated only by a thundering stretch of interstate highway. When I first walked in, he joked that someone should build a tunnel between the two buildings.

As is true for many people in the funeral business, Strommer's gallows humor offsets some of the more somber elements of his work. But he said that talking to someone who was about to die in just a few hours felt unsettling, even to him.

"That plays with your head a little bit," he confessed.

One time, he received a call from a man who wanted to know if he should take the lethal medication while lying down in a body bag or whether he should use a shower curtain. He told Strommer he didn't want to make a mess. Strommer felt amazed at his level of concern. His staff ran a body bag out to the client but assured him that he wouldn't have to place himself in it; they would take care of that. Yet when they arrived for the removal later that day, the client was lying in the bag. He had said goodbye to his family, climbed into the bag, and taken the medication.

"All we had to do was zip him up," said Strommer.

A medically assisted death introduces entirely new possibilities for people to time and choreograph their own death. It imposes a degree of calculability over something that has, until recently, been thought of as fundamentally unknowable, even a mystery. Some find these developments disturbing. Others bristle at the attempt to master death at all. But few are aware of all the barriers someone must overcome to achieve an assisted death.

CHAPTER 5

A Bureaucratic Maze

By the time I arrived at Providence Hospital in Northeast Portland, the rain had soaked through my leather boots and matted my hair. I peeled off my rain pants, stuffed them into my backpack, and locked my bike to a pole. Derianna had told me to meet her on the seventh floor of the cancer ward so I could witness her intake exam of Henry, an eighty-nine-year-old patient who wanted to initiate his application for an assisted death. Henry had been pleading with his social worker to help qualify him, but as a member of a Catholic hospice that doesn't participate in the law, her hands were tied. She had passed his request on to End of Life Choices Oregon to see if someone could talk over Henry's options with him.

As I wandered through a labyrinth of dead-end hallways, I couldn't find a single person to point me to the cancer ward, so I returned to the front desk to ask for directions. For a second, I hesitated. Assisted deaths never take place inside hospitals, and I wasn't sure how staff felt about visitors dropping by to discuss this possibility with their patients. The primary purpose of the modern hospital is to prevent death—not to facilitate it. I felt oddly conspiratorial traipsing up and down the halls of this ghostly Catholic hospital, trying to locate a patient who sought to hasten his death.

I finally got up the nerve to ask the receptionist for directions. It turned out I was in the wrong building. When I rode up to the seventh floor, it was just me and a crumpled-up, purple latex glove that sat discarded in the corner of the elevator, a remnant of the human inter-actions that take place in this clinical space. I found a seat in the wide, fluorescent hallway across from Henry's room.

Minutes later, I watched a tall, portly figure amble toward me. Derianna was without her cane today, and her limp looked more pronounced than usual, her hips stiff. As I saw her inch closer, her playful blue eyes lit up with the spark of recognition. I thought again how steadfast her commitment to this work was—coming up on twenty years—when she had her own infirmities to contend with.

Derianna asked me to wait outside the door while she checked with Henry to see if he was all right with my sitting in on their consultation. It would just be the three of us. He had no objections, and I entered and pulled up a chair next to Derianna, flanking Henry on his right side, his good side, so that he would be able to hear me. Derianna knew from his social worker that Henry was hard of hearing and that glaucoma in both eyes had made him almost completely blind. But I wasn't prepared for him to look as frail as he did. He lay in bed with his bony chest exposed, his ribs showing through his hospital gown, his arms covered in bruises and bandages. A catheter stuck out from underneath his blanket. As Derianna muted the TV, I took Henry's hand in mine and introduced myself. His skin was thin as a fine leather glove.

"Tell me why you think I have come to visit you today," Derianna began.

I had seen this verbal dance many times. Volunteers who work with clients usually won't raise the option of an assisted death unless the patient brings it up first. They want to ensure that someone isn't swayed by the power of suggestion. Derianna's question was open-ended on purpose.

"To help me die with dignity," Henry said, offering her a toothless smile. His voice was unexpectedly soft.

Derianna pressed his hand. Her goal for today was to figure out if Henry could theoretically qualify for Oregon's assisted dying law. Before she and her team would try to find two doctors who would examine him, she needed to be sure he was a viable candidate. She hadn't yet seen his medical chart, and she wasn't certain if he met the primary criterion for an assisted death: a terminal illness that put him within six months of the end of his life. His social worker had given her some bare bones notes about him, but they weren't enough for her to get a clear picture.

Derianna knew that, about two years ago, Henry was diagnosed with lymphoma. For a while, he had received radiation treatment, but she didn't know whether that was meant to be palliative only or whether it had purged the cancer. Seven months ago, Henry was admitted to home hospice care. His admission to hospice would indicate that he was nearing the end of his life, but sometimes patients are admitted to hospice without a clear-cut prognosis. Some physicians aren't willing or able to say that a patient has six months or less to live, but they might still enroll them in hospice.

Derianna got out a notepad and launched into her fact-finding mission. An intake visit required her to become a sleuth, she had told me a while back. Figuring out a patient's unique medical and social situation could feel like a treasure hunt without a map.

"Besides the cancer, do you have any other terminal conditions?" Derianna asked, her eyes moving back and forth between Henry's face and the whiteboard she had just discovered across the room. The board listed his medications and the names of his clinicians. She scribbled down the information, her gaze still fixed on Henry. He said he wasn't sure.

"Are you in any pain right now?" She tried another tactic. Perhaps his pain could be indicative of another underlying illness.

"Just from my fall," Henry replied.

In the past six months, Henry had had two falls. His most recent one was bad—it was what landed him in the hospital a week ago. His nephew, an arborist who lived with him and was his primary caregiver, had to call firefighters to pick him off the floor.

Derianna nodded and asked him what medications he was taking. She couldn't be sure that the whiteboard was correct.

"Steroids," he said. "For pumping iron," he added with a mischievous smirk. Henry lifted his battered arms in a slow upward motion. Derianna guffawed. She loved working with people who had a sense of humor.

Derianna ran through more questions. Had someone entered

Henry's request for assisted dying into his medical chart? It isn't enough for a physician to record talking to a patient about assisted dying in general terms. The chart needs to state explicitly that a patient expressed to a physician, not a nurse or social worker, their desire to use the law. If Henry's request had been documented in such unequivocal terms, it might count as his first oral request, which would jump-start the clock on the fifteen-day waiting period mandated by the law.

Henry couldn't say. He had never seen his chart, and he wasn't sure what his doctors had written down. Sometimes patients think they have started the clock, only to learn months later that their request had not been officially recorded. In his time as a prescribing physician, Charles Blanke had met countless patients who had told their family doctor months before that they wanted to use the law and who thought that stating this had initiated their waiting period. But physicians have to follow a formal checklist for such a request to be legitimate legally.

"A first formal request has to include specific language and pieces from that checklist," Blanke explained. "And I will just tell you, unless they know about the list, most physicians don't bring up all these points during a routine clinic appointment. So the request doesn't count. And as you can imagine, the patient gets angry, and I feel terrible, right? But we can't bend the law."

Following their first oral request, a patient must complete a written request and locate two witnesses willing to sign it (one of whom can neither be a relative nor heir to their estate). Next, they must find two physicians—one acting in an attending role, the other as a consultant—to independently examine them and certify that their terminal condition gives them a reasonable life expectancy of no more than six months. Once the waiting period is over, and assuming a patient checked all the boxes until that point, they have to reiterate to their attending physician their wish to move ahead. Henry stood just at the very beginning of this protocol.

Typically, Derianna would try to get Henry's own doctors to qualify him for the law—they knew him and his medical history the best. Besides, the volunteer doctors who work for her organization are a precious resource that she only taps when a patient's own doctors refuse to participate. But because of Providence's unyielding policy against assisted dying, Derianna already knew she would need to recruit two volunteer doctors to evaluate Henry. Before she could ask them to see him, she would have to review his medical records to make sure he had a terminal diagnosis. She had Henry sign a form that would authorize hospice to release his records to her organization.

Later, Derianna would explain that her questions for Henry also served a secondary purpose. She was doing a mini mental exam to see if Henry was mentally cogent. Did he know his medical history? Was he aware what he was asking for? If a patient suffers from a mental illness or degenerative condition that affects their decision-making capacity, their case has to be referred to a mental health expert. It could take weeks to get an appointment with a psychiatrist, so she wanted to be prepared.

In the midst of our conversation, a nurse came by to check on Henry. She asked him if he needed anything. A juice box? He shook his head. Wait, he did have one request, he signaled.

"Don't let these two ladies leave," he told her, his smile so wide it turned his beady eyes into slits. The nurse threw him a tender glance and left the room. Henry told us that he had no complaints about the care he had received at the hospital so far. His nurses came by regularly to turn him and massage his feet and back. Still, his mind was made up.

"I just want to sleep permanently," he told Derianna now, his voice low and emphatic.

"I understand," she said and gently stroked his forearm. She told Henry that qualifying him for an assisted death wouldn't be possible without a definitive terminal diagnosis.

Henry pressed his lips together and turned his head away from her. He was crying.

For a few seconds, no one said anything. I felt tears pooling in my eyes and stared down at my boots. I had always been moved by seeing older men cry, and seeing this man plead for Derianna's help tore at my heart.

"I can't be sure yet," she spoke softly, still maintaining her composure. "My first priority will be for you to get well enough to leave this hospital."

Before Derianna dedicated herself to her volunteer role full-time, she had spent years as a home hospice and community nurse, trying to keep high-risk elders out of nursing homes and reduce the time they spent in hospitals after a medical event. "People heal better in their own homes," she once told me. "Remove them from their environment and they're lost. They don't know how to act, they don't know how to access the food they like, and they can't sleep."

It was clear that Henry couldn't go home. His two falls had made it plain that his nephew could no longer handle Henry's care by himself. Henry never married and he had no children. Derianna had something else in mind: with the help of his hospice team, she would try to move Henry out of the hospital and into an assisted living facility, where he could continue to receive around-the-clock care while he recuperated.

Then she brought up another option for Henry to consider. She thought he might be a candidate for VSED—voluntary stopping of eating and drinking—which involves a dying patient's deliberate cessation of food and drink. In the last three years, Derianna had supported ten families whose loved one had chosen this path. But the process can be arduous for patients and caregivers alike, taking ten to fourteen days from beginning to end. Because patients become so weak from a lack of food and water, they are at an increased risk of falling. They must be supervised twenty-four hours a day and rotated frequently to avoid bedsores. Most hospitals aren't allowed or even equipped to provide this kind of care, so Henry would have to wait until he was discharged.

Derianna rose to her feet. She told Henry she would try her best to help him. He thanked her and we said goodbye.

As we walked to the parking garage, my arm substituting for her cane, Derianna told me what would come next. She would submit the request to obtain his medical records, reach out to two of her organization's physicians to see if one could come by to examine him, and work with Henry's social worker to get him into an assisted living facility. If Henry managed to qualify for the law, and once a physician wrote his prescription, he would need to find a pharmacy willing to fill his script.

And if his insurance didn't cover the cost of the medication, he would have to figure out how to pay for the drugs. For some patients, spending even seven hundred dollars for the cheaper of two available drug cocktails amounts to serious financial hardship, wiping out any savings they have left. Henry would then need to find a place to die, a facility that didn't have a policy against assisted dying on their premises—unless his nephew was willing to offer up his house. Derianna was committed to supporting Henry each step of the way. But she had six other clients on her roster that week, so she would have to work overtime.

On my ride home, as the rain pelted my skin, my mind returned to the moment when Henry had turned his face away from us. His quiet urgency to be released from this life haunted me, bringing tears back to my eyes. None of the assisted deaths I had attended had affected me quite like this. Maybe it was because those patients had succeeded in their quest to end their life, and their relief was so palpable. Henry didn't have any of that relief yet. For now, he would have to persevere and trust that Derianna would come through for him.

I got off my bike and walked the rest of the way, trying to untangle my thoughts. Then I stepped into a grocery store to pick up a few things.

"What have you been up to today?" the cashier asked as he rang me up.

I went to the hospital to watch someone try to help a patient die, I thought.

"Not much," I said and swiped my card.

———————————

Pursuing an assisted death is fraught with obstacles. To avail themselves of their state's assisted dying law, patients must navigate a maze of legal requirements, bureaucratic procedures, and religious pushback. Maneuvering through this process would be confusing and daunting if you were young and healthy—for someone like Henry, pushing ninety and in the throes of serious illness, it can quickly become unmanageable.

Most people who are caught in the turmoil of terminal illness have little bandwidth to take on the logistical and emotional costs of figuring out how to qualify for assisted dying. Preparing for death and coming to terms with it are difficult enough without that added burden. Many patients rely on home visits by physicians because they are too sick to go to a doctor's office, and even a small delay in their application may slam shut their window for using the law. It's all too easy to become discouraged and give up.

Because of all these challenges, a cadre of trained volunteers has helped support patients and families in their pursuit of an assisted death since the early days of the law. In the Pacific Northwest, volunteers from End of Life Choices Oregon and End of Life Washington act as a bridge between patients and the medical system. They know which physicians are willing to see patients, which pharmacies stock the necessary medications, and what methods work best to dilute the caustic taste of life-ending medication. Volunteers can connect indigent patients to resources to defray the price of the drugs, and they have established a small network of assisted living facilities and private Airbnbs that are willing to host patients for their death. Patients and families find the two organizations online, or they are referred by their physician or hospice. Most feel deeply grateful not to be left alone during such an extraordinary time.

If their presence is requested, which it frequently is, volunteers accompany dying patients and their loved ones on their chosen day. Volunteers typically attend a death in a team of two—one person focused on the patient, the other on the family—unless a physician is also present (in which case only one volunteer goes out). They are prepared to handle complications that may arise during an assisted death and can reassure family members along the way, telling them what to expect at each turn. Their expertise frees families up to focus on being emotionally present with their loved one rather than worrying about procedural issues (like keeping the correct time intervals between the different drugs a patient has to ingest). Most volunteers can recognize death's telltale signs much better than families can, and they ensure that families follow proper protocol after the death. They also act as a resource for families long afterward, debriefing with the bereaved and pointing them to resources to cope with their grief.

There is one additional, delicate task families are often glad to outsource to volunteers: preparing the life-ending medication. Though families may morally support their loved one's decision to hasten their death, the idea of physically assembling their lethal cocktail puts some ill at ease. Linda Jensen, a volunteer for End of Life Choices Oregon, explained one reason behind that reluctance.

"Family members don't want to open the capsules," she said. "They're perfectly capable of opening them, of mixing up the medicine. It's not rocket science. But they don't want to be that agent. They don't want to be the person that in any way facilitated the actual death."

Since late 2018, when Seconal disappeared from pharmacy shelves due to a stock out, volunteers no longer have to open one hundred capsules of Seconal to assemble the medicine. But even the new drug protocols require the mixing of three to four different medications that arrive in separate bottles. Families routinely report being terrified they might do something wrong, even with printed instructions from the pharmacy. During the COVID-19 pandemic, when volunteers and physicians had to move their services online, families' roles suddenly shifted from supportive witness to active facilitator. To enable their loved one to die, families had to step up and prepare the medication themselves—with volunteers coaching them over Zoom.

In the hours I spent with volunteers during monthly meetings, trainings, and interviews, several things struck me: almost all volunteers were women, most were retired, and many had spent their careers working in medical settings as nurses or social workers. They were drawn to the work because they had seen the benefits of an assisted death firsthand or because they wished that option had been available to a loved one they watched die.

Andrea Sigetich fell into the first category. A sensible, can-do woman in her sixties, she accompanied her husband, Beryl, on his path to an assisted death in 2016. Seven years prior, Beryl had received a diagnosis of chronic obstructive pulmonary disease (COPD), and he had been on portable oxygen for the last five. For the couple, it was out of the question that Beryl would try to have a "natural" death. They had researched what it's like to die from COPD, and they knew they weren't going to take that route.

"It's probably worse than most cancers," Andrea said when we sat down in her ranch house near Bend, the scent of sagebrush wafting in through the open windows. "Basically, you suffocate." Her husband was already on morphine for his pain through hospice, but he disliked the sensation of being drugged. Wanting to manage his own destiny, he kept fastidious track of his morphine intake on a five-by-eight-inch index card.

Beryl ran into unforeseen delays with his request for assisted dying. His internist of ten years had promised she would serve as his prescriber, even though she had no prior experience with the law. She began sifting through websites, forms, and protocols to figure out the steps she needed to take. Every few days, she would share her progress notes with Andrea, who had started doing research on her own. At the time, neither of them had any idea about the sequence of requests, the fifteen-day waiting period, or the requirement for a second physician.

"Everybody in Oregon knows that we have this law," Andrea told me. "But nobody has a clue how it works." Her voice rang with disbelief.

As the weeks ticked on, Beryl's decline was rapid. One evening, as Andrea helped him to the bathroom, he turned to her and said, "It's supposed to be death with dignity. I don't have any dignity left." That was when Andrea wished they had the prescription in hand. But she was still trying to figure out which pharmacy could even fill it. Beryl's internist had only just taken his first oral request. Over the following two weeks, Beryl deteriorated further. When Andrea asked him a question, he would sometimes take ten minutes to respond. She sensed that he was actively dying.

Beryl's medications arrived through FedEx from Portland on a Wednesday afternoon. That evening, he took the lethal drugs—he could not wait a second longer. Andrea mixed the medicine and poured it into his best scotch glass. Ten minutes after drinking the dose, Beryl fell unconscious. Andrea kept talking to him, and she kept his oxygen on in case he needed it. Over the next forty minutes, his breathing got slower. Then it stopped.

"It was so damn peaceful," she said.

For Andrea, the biggest difference between waiting to "let things take their course" and Beryl's desire for an assisted death was that she didn't have to feel so helpless in the process. Supporting his death gave her a sense of control in a time of intense uncertainty. The day after our talk, she sent me an email to make sure I understood why she had helped Beryl die.

"As a caregiver, I helped him live while he was living," she wrote. "I helped him eat, manage his morphine and his other medications, use the bathroom, shower, and communicate with his kids and his nurse. And then I helped him die when it was time to die—something he so wanted and was ready for. It was a profound expression of my love for this man, to assist him in the journey he must take, even though two years later I remain immersed in grief and sorrow."

One and a half years after his death, Andrea began volunteering for

End of Life Choices Oregon. She wanted to prevent others from having to download random forms from the internet and not know how the process worked. If she could save other families from floundering the way she did while racing against the clock, she would try.

Other volunteers fell into the work for opposite reasons. "Most people who are in this work have watched some pretty bad deaths," Derianna told me one day as we were driving to a volunteer meeting on Portland's West Side. "Some horrific, painful, excruciating, complicated deaths." They figured there must be another way to die, perhaps a better way.

Derianna was no exception. When she was thirty-five, her father took a gun to his head under an oak tree he had planted with her twenty years prior at their home in rural Ohio. He had been in chronic, unmanaged pain her entire life. Shortly after she was born, her father had fallen off a cliff while inspecting his Texan dude ranch on horseback. He shattered his hip, back, knees, and ankles and soon began self-medicating with alcohol. Derianna wasn't there to witness his death, but her mother was.

Two years later, her mother took her life. Derianna called it a covert suicide. She had long worried that her mother wouldn't have the emotional capacity to survive on her own after her husband's death—as contentious as their marriage had been, it had also been codependent. One morning, her mother stood in the bathroom, brushing her long, blond hair until it was full of electricity. Absentmindedly, she lit a cigarette, and her hair caught on fire. What started as an accident turned into something more intentional. Instead of calling for help, her mother doused the fire and, with massive burns on her face and chest, climbed into bed and started drinking liquor and eating pills.

Derianna believed that her mother wanted to die—she had always been a beauty queen and proud of her good looks, and she was never going to adapt to being so disfigured. Derianna's two siblings eventually called an ambulance, which rushed their mother to the intensive care burn unit. By the next morning, she had flatlined. Physicians declared her brain dead and put her on a ventilator. Derianna flew in from Texas to hold counsel with her siblings on what to do. As distraught as she was over losing her mother, she knew that her mother was never going to regain consciousness, and she begged her siblings to let her go. She felt indignant that her mother was being kept alive against her wishes. Two weeks later, on Christmas day, her siblings agreed to take their mother off life support.

"Those were the hardest seventeen days of my life," Derianna remembered.

Her parents' violent deaths shook Derianna to the core. But her response was different from what one might expect of someone in her situation. Rather than turning away from death, she turned toward it—not immediately, but years later. If she was ever going to properly process her trauma, she thought, she needed to better understand death. A decade after her mother's suicide, Derianna went into hospice nursing.

"I really wanted to kill that dragon, the dragon of being afraid of death. It was full frontal: take your biggest fear and face it head on."

Years prior, she had earned a nursing degree from Ohio State University and worked as a nurse in six states. Since settling down in Texas with her husband, she had become certified as a midwife, specializing in home births. At the time, husbands weren't allowed to attend hospital births and cesarean sections were quickly becoming the norm. After her parents' deaths, she felt that it was time to shift her focus.

Initially, Derianna felt apprehensive about being with people who were dying. But she soon came to love hospice nursing. It allowed her to work with people in their own homes and share in life's most meaningful moments, just as she had done as a midwife. Caring for people at the end of life gave her a glimpse into the depths of human grace and resilience. Many of the farewells she witnessed were so loving, they taught her that death didn't have to be inevitably tragic.

In 1998, a few months after Oregon had passed the Death with Dignity Act, Derianna took a job as a community nurse for high-risk elders in Newport on the Oregon coast. Having lived in Texas for thirty-two years and watching her marriage disintegrate, she felt hungry for a shake-up. Within a month of her arrival, she met a volunteer from Compassion in Dying during a water aerobics class at the local pool. The idea of an organization dedicated to helping people die felt like a revelation to her, and one month later, she started as a volunteer herself.

"And I've been doing it ever since," she said and smiled. Twenty years later, she was the oldest and longest serving assisted dying volunteer in Oregon.

When I first met Derianna, she had just returned from a conference on conscious dying—the idea that people who are close to death and in the right state of mind can will themselves to die. She thought it explained why people sometimes die the day after a big event, like a birthday or an anniversary. They wait for the occasion, and then they die the next day.

"That's how I want to go," said Derianna as I sank into her plush sofa cushions. "I want to see if I can just let go and die."

If it were up to her, dying patients wouldn't have to be at the mercy of any medication to end their lives. Because even if someone failed to get a prescription or missed their window for taking it, she believed they should be able to have a self-determined death—by declining food and drink, for example. "My job, as I see it, is to help people die the way they want to, not to push the medicine but to let them know how strong and powerful they are."

Over the next three years, I spent countless afternoons on her couch, sipping tea and devouring her crackers and stories, enveloped by a thick cloud of eucalyptus that spread from her diffusers. We went to library readings and backyard concerts together, simmered in her backyard hot tub, and once we crashed an "Italian Cruise" party at an assisted living facility so Derianna could speak with management about allowing assisted deaths on their premises.

The times I attended a death with her, Derianna was a quiet, clear-headed presence. Dressed formally for the occasion, she took her cues from the patient and family, offered advice when it seemed helpful, and remained in the background the rest of the time. She thought the best thing she could do for someone who is dying is bring positive, serene energy to the room. But she also believed that someone could accomplish an assisted death without a volunteer there. When she sensed a desire for privacy, she coached the patient and family on how to prepare the medication and stepped back. And she made herself available on the day of the death, her phone charged in case they called.

One day, after I had known her for a year, Derianna pulled down her blouse to show me the three-letter, bold-faced tattoo that adorned her upper chest: DNR—do not resuscitate. She knew that DNR tattoos aren't legally binding, but she got a big kick out of hers.

"I'm thinking of putting my POLST number underneath," she said and winked.

A physician's order for life-sustaining treatment (POLST) is a form that details a person's wishes regarding medical interventions at the end of life. In the course of her career, Derianna had become critical of aggressive, life-prolonging measures. She believed that, more often than not, high-tech interventions close to death only compound someone's suffering rather than add quality time to their life.

"I think that we keep people alive artificially in this country. We overmedicate and overtreat and overprescribe procedures. I would like to think that when my time is ready, I'll know, and I'll be glad to go. I have an expiration date, and I want to honor that."

Talking to Derianna about death and dying became as commonplace as talking about the weather. She had spent more than half her life breaking down the taboos and barriers that kept people from engaging meaningfully with their own mortality. As a hospice nurse and later as a volunteer, Derianna had shepherded hundreds of people over the threshold between life and death. And it was assisted deaths specifically that left an indelible impression on her.

"I got to see a window into the other side. I could watch patients let go and be at peace and know they were free from suffering, free from angst. The first time I watched an assisted death, I thought, *Oh my God, it's just like a good birth*. It felt just like a good birth."

Her exposure therapy worked: in the autumn of her life, she had made friends with death.

"I have no fear now, no fear whatsoever," she told me, an impish grin on her lips. "In fact, I look forward to it."

Derianna had already researched different disposition methods, and she liked the idea of her ashes being planted as a tree. But she had problems with traditional cremation because of the fuel expenditure. Either way, she knew she didn't want to ship her body anywhere after her death.

"One of my daughters wants my body buried on our ranch in Texas, but it was hot as hell when I lived there, and I would rather not travel posthumously."

For all her convictions around honoring and supporting someone's desire to die, the magnitude of that choice was never lost on her.

"This is a daunting decision, and it deserves to be thought out carefully. People need to be absolutely sure they're ready to go. And they need to know it's okay for them to change their mind and to call us when they're ready."

Henry was ready. With the help of his social worker, Derianna had managed to move him into a nursing home where he continued to convalesce from his fall. A week later, two volunteer physicians from End of Life Choices Oregon came by to examine him and certified his eligibility for an assisted death based on a life-threatening diagnosis of lymphatic cancer. Because his nursing home had a policy against assisted dying, Henry's nephew offered to have his uncle die at his house. Derianna attended the death, along with a dozen of Henry's friends.

"He was loved by so many," she said. "It was a beautiful death."

CHAPTER 6

Medical Gatekeepers

Physicians who work with terminally ill patients sometimes find themselves in a bind. On one hand, their professional ethos tells them to preserve and possibly extend life. On the other hand, they have a basic duty to relieve suffering. But what if relieving a patient's suffering means helping them die?

During his early years in family medicine, David Grube witnessed the gruesome death of one of his patients. He says it still haunts him forty years later. Jerry, a man in his fifties, was suffering from bladder cancer that had metastasized to his bones and left him in uncontrollable pain. With his life expectancy measured in weeks, Jerry had enrolled in hospice. On one of Grube's days off, he got a call from Jerry's son, who lived just around the corner from him in Philomath, Oregon. He asked Grube to come over to the house, and quickly.

"There's something wrong with Dad," he said.

"And it's just a couple hundred yards, so I went over to his house,"

Grube recalled. "The TV in the bedroom was on so loud you could hear it from the street. I went into the room and Jerry was sitting in a chair between the twin beds in their bedroom with a shotgun in his lap and nothing above his neck—everything on the ceiling. This was the worst experience of my clinical practicing. It really impacted my whole psyche. This can't ever—this is the worst way."

Jerry's death was a turning point in Grube's career. Having had no legal ways of assisting Jerry to ease his anguish, Grube felt he had failed him as a doctor. Years later, when assisted dying became legal in Oregon, Grube was one of two dozen physicians in the law's second year to prescribe life-ending medication to a patient—at a time when prescribers risked being ostracized by their colleagues and dumped by their patients. In 2015, three years after he retired, Grube became the medical director for Compassion and Choices, a national organization that advocates for patients' rights to determine the terms of their own death.

Yet for all his dedication to the cause, Grube thinks it's unfortunate that the right-to-die movement has claimed the term "dignity" for itself. There are many ways to have a dignified death, he says. An assisted death is just one of them.

"Who defines dignity? It's defined by the dying person," Grube told me. "I don't define their dignity. Only they can define their dignity, so if they want to be in the ICU on a breathing machine with an IV and catheters—if that's what they want, that's dignity for them."

Despite some of their personal differences, physicians at the helm of assisted dying see the right to die as an integral part of practicing good medicine. For them, medicine's obligation to alleviate suffering doesn't stop once disease takes over—it extends until a patient draws their last breath.

———————

Some physicians are prepared to help patients pursue an assisted death, but many more are not. In 2020, 142 physicians prescribed medications under Oregon's Death with Dignity Act—out of 6,200 physicians in the state.[1] The Oregon law allows physicians to opt out of being involved in an assisted death, with no legal obligation to refer a patient elsewhere. As a result, some patients spend weeks or months trying to find a physician willing to see them. By the time they finally do, they sometimes burst into tears.

Physicians are the ones who ultimately decide which patients meet the conditions of the law and which do not. In their role as medical gatekeepers, they are charged with interpreting and enforcing the letter of the law—to the best of their ability and conscience.

Charles Blanke, who runs a research oncology unit at the Oregon Health and Science University, has written the most prescriptions for assisted dying of any physician in Oregon. He believes that doctors have an ethical obligation to not desert their patients at the end of life. And yet, he says, it happens all the time.

"Usually, a patient's doctor will say, 'I don't do it. I don't know anybody who does. Good luck with that.' I think it's a shame that the doctor a patient has had for seventeen years won't help them. But they won't, and I will."

Blanke thinks that enabling a very sick patient to die is the opposite of doing harm—it's a compassionate thing to do. He knows that many of his hospital colleagues aren't necessarily opposed to assisted dying on moral grounds. But they don't want to be directly responsible for causing a patient's death—even if they have stopped pacemakers, withdrawn life support, or given permission to dial up a patient's morphine drip many times before.

Blanke doesn't hide his services. But patients have to be savvy to find him. "And they have to be persistent," he added, his high forehead creased with concern. "Or else they're screwed. If you get somebody who's relatively poor or homeless or who doesn't have computer access or a phone—they're going to have some trouble."

Though Blanke's speech was naturally fast, it barely kept up with the pace of his thoughts. Talking to the doctor felt like entering a high-stakes ping-pong match: if you could bounce the ball back quickly and adeptly, he would let you mine the depth of his brain. His animated restlessness had caused him to develop insomnia, but it's also made him a fastidious physician. He didn't take the responsibility of helping someone die lightly.

"It's a pretty profound thing to give somebody a medication that you know will end their life," he said, folding his hands behind his head as if to grasp the sheer weight of that burden.

When a patient was too ill to see him, Blanke stuffed himself into his black leather jacket, jumped on his motorcycle, and paid them a house call. Unlike most of his colleagues, he had the luxury of time: his research unit brought in millions of dollars in grants each year, decreasing the financial pressure he felt to cycle patients through his practice in fifteen-minute increments. If he wanted to, he could spend four hours discussing a patient's end-of-life concerns.

Opponents of assisted dying often accuse patients who seek an assisted death of "doctor shopping"—of leapfrogging from doctor to doctor until they find someone to sign off on their request. But when faced with physicians who refuse to even schedule an appointment, patients quickly reach an impasse.

When she used to work with assisted dying patients, Ellen Bartlett, a retired internal medicine doctor from Washington State, routinely trekked from Seattle across the Cascade Mountains to the eastern part of the state to see patients because their own doctors would not. She said she went to more trailer homes than mansions. Bartlett echoed the sentiment of her Oregon colleagues: physicians have a moral responsibility to not abandon their patients.

"Some oncologists treat these patients; they take them through really horrible treatment, it makes patients miserable, and when they don't have anything else to throw at them, they say, 'Well, sorry, go get your affairs in order and we'll see you.' They abandon them. And I think that's wrong. Doctors are more comfortable with pushing and pushing and doing everything they can to keep people going. But I think most of us aren't very comfortable with death."

Telling a patient they are dying isn't just uncomfortable. It means accepting the limits of medicine's seemingly infinite ability to "do something" and transitioning into a different kind of care. In *Being Mortal*, Atul Gawande describes his reluctance to admit to one of his cancer patients that she had run out of treatment options. Doing so would have meant acknowledging that she was dying. "I even raised with her the possibility that an experimental therapy could work against both her cancers, which was sheer fantasy," Gawande writes. "Discussing a fantasy was easier—less emotional, less explosive, less prone to misunderstanding—than discussing what was happening before my eyes."[2]

But even if a doctor is comfortable talking about death, they often run into logistical constraints. An end-of-life consult takes three to four times longer than a regular appointment, and many physicians can't budget that much time for one patient. Physicians with no previous exposure to assisted dying fear having to deal with a mountain of bureaucracy, even though the forms are fairly straightforward. Others worry about losing their license if they make a mistake or being shamed by colleagues for showing support for a law that remains controversial, even among physicians. To this day, the American Medical Association opposes assisted dying, arguing that the practice (which they refer to as "physician-assisted suicide") "is fundamentally incompatible with the physician's role as healer."[3]

For all these reasons, many doctors who serve as prescribing or consulting physicians are retired and volunteer their services free of charge. Neil Martin, Ken's physician, retired from family medicine in 2015, but he kept his license to volunteer. For Martin, the emotional impact of helping a patient die requires a good deal of downtime. His retirement has given him the space to take on emotionally charged work and not feel depleted by the end of the day.

"It's so much harder during clinical practice to shift gears emotionally when dealing with a dying person," Martin said, his voice mild and measured. "I think most doctors are exhausted at the end of the day with all the decisions they have had to make, that adding the emotional burden of addressing death for someone feels too demanding."

A few times a week, Martin operated a laser at a tattoo removal clinic in inner-city Portland that caters to an indigent population, erasing painful past reminders of prison, domestic violence, and gang affiliations. He jokes that it's part of his commitment to the beautification of Portland. In reality, the work fit in with his larger philosophy of not allowing someone's past—their choices, crimes, or illnesses—to dictate their prospects for the future.

Working with assisted dying patients reminded Martin of why he had entered the field of medicine so many years ago. "You're stepping into a role that has a profound impact on a person's life. And they're looking to you with great hope—with great expectation—that you will work with them for the death they want. So much of medicine grinds through on a day-to-day basis, and you lose the emotional connection. But assisted dying gets back to the core of why I became a physician: to do that relief of suffering."

Martin first became involved as a prescribing physician in 2009. His parents had both belonged to the Hemlock Society in hopes of being able to end their lives when their time had come. His father, a German immigrant, passed away in a hospital in California in 1996 before any assisted dying laws had been enacted. His mother, who had emigrated from China in her early twenties, moved up to join Martin and his wife in Portland. Throughout his mother's decline over the next nineteen years, she held on to her desire to die if and when her life became intolerable to her. In 2015, Martin's mother did qualify for an assisted death and took the medication with her son at her bedside. He held her hand as she passed.

As physicians, Blanke and Martin were used to escorting their patients through the vagaries of disease, glissading from one treatment cycle to the next. And they remained involved after all treatment options had been exhausted. For these physicians, ensuring a humane death was as much a part of being a good doctor as saving someone's life.

When he first began prescribing life-ending medication under the law, Nick Gideonse made a pact with himself: he would never take the initiative to suggest assisted dying to a patient. He had been in family medicine for years, accompanying patients from birth to death. But even when a colleague referred a patient to him and his schedule read "Death with Dignity consultation," Gideonse stuck to his rule.

Sitting in a busy Portland coffee shop, his untamed, grizzled curls gainsaying his youthful looks, Gideonse put down his cup and told me point-blank: "I am never going to suggest that you end your life." For a second, I wondered if we had any eavesdroppers and what they were thinking. "You're going to *ask* me, and you're not going do it in a euphemism either."

In his clinic, the conversation usually went something like this:

"What are you here for today?" Gideonse would ask, leaning his tall frame back in his chair and listening intently as his patient grasped for words.

"You're going to help me pass to the other side," the patient might respond.

Gideonse shook his head and set his palms down flat on the table.

"No," Gideonse would counter. "Tell me exactly what you're hoping I will do or what we'll do together."

Unless the patient said they were seeking a lethal prescription to help them die, the conversation would go no further. Gideonse knew that not raising assisted dying as an option might prevent some patients from being aware that it existed and from making use of it. But if it meant ensuring that those who did use it were doing so freely, he was willing to pay that price. As a physician, he was sharply aware of the cultural authority he wielded.

Despite their willingness to discuss assisted dying, prescribing physicians rarely bring it up as an option to their patients. Like Gideonse, many worry about the coercive effect of offering assisted dying unprompted. Physicians don't want to inadvertently push patients toward the law or undercut patients' belief that—as their doctors—they would do everything in their power to care for them.

Gideonse and his colleagues spend much of the initial meeting exploring why a patient is requesting assistance in dying and whether they have thought about other options. This is when patients open up about their inmost fears: about losing their sense of self, about having nothing but bad days ahead of them, about dying in pain, about facing an undignified ending. Gideonse then tries to figure out how to address these concerns outside an assisted dying framework. Sometimes he gets the patient's whole family into the room to brainstorm together.

"I am really trying very hard to meet and discern a patient's deepest needs and look for alternative ways to meet their needs beyond a lethal prescription," he said.

Some of that discussion always revolves around hospice. But because the vast majority of patients who use assisted dying laws are already on hospice, it's usually not an option they haven't considered—it's just not enough to relieve their concerns.

His colleague, Charles Blanke, follows a similar tactic. He lays out all the alternatives and makes sure the patient has a complete under-standing of what the end of their life might look like, with or without using the law.

"I don't judge the quality of their reason, but I do believe that if they're suffering from something that I can take away, then maybe they won't do it, and maybe they will enjoy their last six months," Blanke told me. "So I do feel that obligation to dig deeper, and I pursue that pretty aggressively. But once it's clear that their suffering is not going to go away, in their opinion—not my opinion—then I one hundred percent support their decision."

For Blanke, a patient's right to decide routinely outweighed his impulse for medical paternalism, even if he didn't agree with a patient's personal reasons. His job as a physician, he said, was to outline a patient's choices—the pluses and the minuses, the risks and the benefits—to help someone make the best choice for themselves.

Belief in a patient's right to self-determination was the single most noticeable quality prescribing physicians shared. Contrary to doctors who would coax their patients into doing what they themselves deemed best, these doctors were champions of patient autonomy.

For good reason. The right to die emerged in part as a response to medicine's growing omnipotence. Over the course of the twentieth century, physicians' arsenal for maintaining life on the edges virtually exploded. The increasingly routine use of life support treatments such as feeding tubes and mechanical ventilators in American hospitals prompted patients to protect themselves from futile and aggressive medical interventions—especially at the end of life.

The landmark Karen Ann Quinlan case brought these concerns into sharp focus. A New Jersey woman in her early twenties, Quinlan had fallen into a coma after a night out drinking with her friends in April 1975. She was put on a ventilator and a feeding tube, with little hope for recovery. Over the course of the next year, Quinlan's parents fought for the right to turn off the machines that were keeping their daughter in a persistent vegetative state. In March 1976, the New Jersey Supreme Court ruled that Quinlan's right to refuse treatment was protected by the Constitution's right to liberty and privacy.

By the time of Quinlan's court case, popular confidence in physicians had begun to wane. The medical paternalism of an earlier era had given way to the creeping suspicion that physicians might not always have the best interests of their patients at heart. In Alabama, Black men suffering from syphilis were purposefully left untreated as part of the Tuskegee study, and Black women across America unwittingly underwent forced sterilization. Mounting healthcare costs and the growing specialization of the profession compounded a new sense of physicians as faceless bureaucrats with an agenda of their own.[4] Attempting to hem in medicine's unbridled authority inside a largely private, for-profit health system, right-to-die activists fought to safeguard the rights of dying patients—which, for the longest time, meant gaining the right to *decline* treatment rather than actively expediting death. It wasn't until 1990, with the passage of the federal Patient Self-Determination Act, that patients across America were granted the right to reject medical treatment at the end of life.

The patient-centered approach of prescribing physicians isn't without its limits. One of Grube's patients, who had been diagnosed with diabetes, told him that he wanted to die because he didn't want to face the difficulty of being a diabetic. He asked Grube if he could qualify for an assisted death. Grube refused. He told the patient that his professional integrity rose above the patient's autonomy. Because diabetes is considered a chronic but not inevitably lethal condition—and widely treatable with insulin—Grube couldn't agree to help his patient die.

Just having a conversation with a doctor about assisted dying sometimes puts a patient's mind at ease, and they never initiate the process. Talking about an assisted death typically opens a much broader dialogue about a person's values at the end of life: What do they want to do with the time they have left? Have they filled out an advance directive? Is their will in order? Have they enrolled in hospice? Does their family know about their end-of-life wishes? Given the chance to voice their worries and desires to a caring provider, a patient's urgency to pursue an assisted death occasionally fades away.

When a patient remains undeterred, prescribing physicians turn their attention to one of the thornier parts of their work: to assess whether a patient meets the six-month time frame for terminality required by the law.

Six months might seem like an arbitrary threshold for saying that someone with a terminal illness is close to death. Why does a patient who is within six months qualify for an assisted death but not someone who is seven months or a year away?

When the Oregon Right to Die committee drafted the original bill, they narrowed in on the six-month requirement as a cutoff point because it overlapped with the admission criteria for hospice. A patient must be within six months of the end of their life to be admitted to a hospice service funded by Medicare. There's one big difference: if a physician refers someone to hospice and they outlive their prognosis, there are no consequences. A small minority of patients are on hospice for years. As long as they show continuous decline, they will remain enrolled. But if a physician underestimates the time an assisted dying patient has left, they may cut short a life.

Prescribing physicians like Blanke know that some primary care physicians play it fast and loose with the six-month benchmark for hospice—especially when dealing with an elderly patient with multi-system failure who expresses an interest in hospice.

"The six-month requirement for hospice is the softest requirement you've ever seen," Blanke explained. "I've never seen anybody turned down for hospice, and it's not unusual for somebody to live for eight months, or twelve months, or eighteen months on hospice. And then you say, 'Oh well, I was wrong.' But the problem is, assisted dying is irrevocable. So those six months, they are real. You really have to believe that someone is imminently dying."

For that reason, prescribing physicians cannot rely on existing prognoses for hospice. Besides, even if a patient is already on hospice, they may not have received a specific time frame from their provider. Prescribing physicians must therefore apply their own metrics and criteria to determine if a patient with a serious illness is likely to die within six months. And making that kind of prediction can be daunting—it introduces the possibility for uncertainty and error.

Elizabeth Steiner Hayward, a physician and state senator in Oregon, knows how heavily the responsibility for making a correct prognosis weighs on prescribing physicians and how difficult it is to get it right. She says it sometimes keeps her up at night.

"One of the biggest challenges of any physician is to predict when someone's going to die," she told me. "We're not God."

Steiner Hayward remembered vividly a case from her private clinical practice, when she diagnosed a male patient with stage-four lung cancer. The patient declined treatment, which put him at a life expectancy of three to four months, according to available statistics. His oncologist concurred. But the patient was adamant about walking his daughter down the aisle the following summer. Nine months later, he did, and he died a month after that.

If Steiner Hayward had been asked to assist with his death, she would have determined that he had less than six months to live—when in fact he had ten. What is more typical, however, is that she thinks someone has about a year left, and they are gone within three months. Knowing that she is prone to overshooting helps her feel more comfortable when making a prognosis for a patient who seeks an assisted death. But she errs on the side of caution no matter what.

In *Death Foretold*, sociologist Nicholas Christakis explains why physicians are so hesitant to give a prognosis and why they often overestimate how long a patient has to live. Prognostication, he writes, is "technically difficult and emotionally frightening."[5]

"Physicians [avoid] prognostication…because they [do] not want to deal with its unpleasant aspects or to think about the limits of their ability to change the future. But they also [avoid] it because they [want] to deceive themselves about death, as if in not predicting death they could avoid causing it or witnessing it."[6]

Physicians tend to be overly optimistic about how long a patient has left, especially if they have known someone for a long time. A review of physicians' prognoses for terminally ill cancer patients found that physicians consistently overestimate survival.[7]

To determine how long a patient has left to live, Nick Gideonse does what he calls a "back-of-the-envelope calculation." First, he conducts a physical exam and assesses a patient's caloric and fluid consumption rates. He asks about their weight and appetite. How much are they eating? What's their outtake? Gideonse knows that someone with a draining wound, an active infection, and a low-grade fever is going to consume water and calories quicker than somebody who has a sedentary illness with a slow metabolism, like heart failure. By comparison, someone carrying three liters of water in each leg and another few liters in their abdomen is going to live a lot longer without eating or drinking anything.

Next, he evaluates a patient's physical capacity. How far could they walk a month ago, and how far are they walking now? In his experience, when a cancer patient takes to bed, they rarely have more than a month left; it's a sign of how weak they have become. Gideonse says he doesn't have to be an oncologist to know that the potential complications of immobility—bedsores, infection, pneumonia, blood clots—limit the time a patient has left, even with exceptional care. As the medical director of a high-needs nursing home, he thinks about all a patient's organ systems, not just their tumor. And he couches his degree of certainty in a range.

"If I say one month plus or minus a week, I'm pretty sure that you've got about a month left. If I say six weeks plus or minus ten weeks, I'm really uncertain about the prognosis. But whatever the degree of uncertainty, people are tremendously grateful to have something to work with because they are trying to write their last chapter. I find people almost as grateful for my willingness to stake a bet on their prognosis as they are for the prescription."

Predicting how long someone has left is a bit like forecasting the weather—the closer to the actual date, the more accurate the projection. In fact, it is rare for assisted dying patients to outlive their physicians' prognoses. In 2020, only 3 percent of patients who qualified for an assisted death in Oregon lived past the six-month mark before using the medication.[8]

When prescribing and consulting physicians examine a patient, they supplement their impressions with information from the patient's medical file. Even if their own specialty falls outside the scope of a patient's disease, they have access to prior evaluations by specialists. So even if a gynecologist has to make a prognosis for a cancer patient, she can draw on a wealth of information in the patient's chart. Besides, a prescribing physician will often attempt to find a consulting physician who is an expert on the patient's condition.

Tom Samuels, the pulmonologist who worked with Joe and Anna, has seen hundreds of ALS patients and understands their disease trajectory much better than a nonspecialist would. As a consulting physician, he can determine with a high degree of certainty when they are likely to die, based on a variety of tests that assess their lung function. When Samuels is asked to prognosticate the life span of a patient with COPD, he adds other symptoms to his consideration. Sometimes patients with COPD recover from periods of limited breathing capacity, like those brought on by a bad cold or pneumonia. Before he feels comfortable saying that a COPD patient won't live past six months, Samuels needs three things to be true: the patient is homebound, on oxygen nearly all day long, and so short of breath that they cannot get out of bed. For Samuels, as for his colleagues, there is just no margin for error.

Prescribing physicians have one more box to check before they can qualify someone for assisted dying: a patient must have the mental capacity to make a fully informed, rational decision about their health. If a physician suspects that a patient suffers from a mental illness that might affect their decision-making ability, their case must undergo further scrutiny by a mental health expert. This requirement excludes anyone with substantial cognitive impairment from using the law, such as patients with advanced dementia. The clause is also meant to protect against a patient acting on suicidal ideations in the context of a severe mental illness.

"We know that sixty to seventy percent of people who commit suicide have a mental disorder, particularly severe depression," Linda Ganzini said when we spoke in her office at the Portland Veterans Affairs Medical Center.[9] She is a prominent Oregon psychiatrist who has published extensively on medically assisted deaths. "If we treated the depression, they would make a different choice. But that's just a small subset of people who want assisted dying."

Ganzini readily acknowledges that the screening process for mental disorders is more complicated than assisted dying laws might suggest. Doctors try to evaluate what she calls the "authenticity" of a patient's decision to pursue an assisted death, that is, whether their decision is consistent with their long-term coping strategies. She gave the example of a person having expressed for years their desire to pursue an assisted death if they ever became terminally ill.

Gideonse has developed his own mechanism for assessing if a patient's desire to end their life stems from a place of mental rather than physical pathology. When depressive symptoms are marked on a patient's chart or when the patient has a history of treated depression, he asks one question: "If I had a magic wand, if we did invent the cure that could remove this cancer from your life tomorrow, would you still be pursuing this?"

The patient's response usually makes it clear what the driving force behind their wish to die is. Because if someone says they would still rather die, then Gideonse knows he will request a psychological consult.

Physicians are of course aware that a fatal diagnosis may cause someone to experience profound sadness that their life is ending. Plus, the side effects of a life-threatening disease like cancer—loss of appetite, fatigue, feelings of hopelessness, sleep irregularity—can look exactly like the telltale signs of a major depressive disorder. The challenge for physicians is to figure out whether any of these symptoms indicate a mental disturbance and whether the latter is impairing a patient's judgment. Grube explained the difference:

"You have to start with the fact that one hundred percent of people who are about to die are grieving and sad. If they're happy that they're about to die, that's probably mental illness. But in a major depressive disorder, generally it doesn't just show up willy-nilly when you get terminally ill. It's been going on for many years. If they've been on antidepressants before, that makes me sit up a little straighter and ask harder questions. But if they're really sad because they got liver cancer, wow, they should be. It's horrible."

Signs of depression need not, in and of themselves, raise questions about a patient's decision-making capacity. Depression can be a normal response to an overwhelming crisis, like a patient's loss of functionality.

That doesn't mean that they lose their ability for rational thought. And that's ultimately what physicians need to ascertain.

In practice, physicians rarely encounter patients whose mental status raises red flags. In 2020, Oregon doctors made use of the law's mental health referral clause for just three of the 245 patients who received prescriptions that year.[10] But when physicians do refer a patient, it can leave them deeply conflicted.

One of Blanke's patients had an incurable form of cancer and fell within the six-month rule. Though he qualified for the law on paper, his reasons for wanting to end his life were less conventional. Blanke estimated that his patient had about four months of quality time left before things would take a turn. When he asked him why he wanted to use the law, the patient told him that he didn't have any friends or any quality of life for that matter. He didn't mention his illness at all. And yet he technically was eligible for the law.

"That one was a little challenging for me," said Blanke. "I don't see that very often."

Worried that his patient might be suffering from a depressive disorder, Blanke referred him to a psychiatrist, who determined that his patient was competent and not depressed.

"Or, if he was depressed, it wasn't affecting his competency," Blanke added. In the end, he agreed to write the prescription.

When all is said and done, physicians don't have to agree with the precise reasons behind a patient's decision to die. But they have to ensure that a patient is mentally capable of taking moral responsibility for their choice.

The work of physicians doesn't end once they sit down to write the lethal prescription. They have to figure out which combination of drugs will reliably end someone's life. Physicians have to mobilize the art of medicine—an imperfect art prone to human doubt and error—toward a new science of dying.

CHAPTER 7

The Science of Dying

Most people probably imagine an assisted death, while emotionally difficult, to be technically straightforward: ingest the medication and die. The reality is far more complicated. There is no magic pill that will end a person's life, and physicians aren't taught how to terminate the lives of their patients in medical school—their training is focused entirely on how to keep people alive. Pharmacy textbooks don't offer any direction either. In the absence of any clinical trials or peer-reviewed studies, physicians have had to teach themselves the science of dying. Over the years, they have devised their own drug protocols, sometimes through trial and error.

Lonny Shavelson knows that the pharmacology of assisted dying is still in its infancy. Between 2016 and 2021, the former emergency physician ran Bay Area End of Life Options, a private Berkeley practice specializing in medically assisted deaths. Shavelson and his team stood at the bedside of over two hundred patients as they took the lethal medication. And he has faced his fair share of riddles.

"Why did Prince die in an elevator after taking a small dose of fentanyl when we are giving our patients huge doses of medications and they're not dying in an hour?" he posited when we first spoke in 2018, his pointed face framed by a salt-and-pepper beard and round spectacles. "They're dying in five or six hours."

Since then, Shavelson and his colleagues across the country have been getting closer to unlocking the science of dying, but he says some work remains.

Shavelson is something of a renegade in the assisted dying world. When California enacted the End of Life Option Act in 2016, he launched his own private practice focused solely on patients considering an assisted death. At the time, medical systems and university hospitals were scrambling to put their own protocols into place. Twenty years prior, Shavelson had written a stirring book, *A Chosen Death*, on his experience accompanying five patients who sought out an assisted death underground, prior to legalization. When the California law passed, he saw the chance to assist in the rollout and leave his mark. Energetic and unafraid of controversy, he became fixated on cracking the code behind the science of dying.

There are many pharmacological complications that can thwart a person's desire for a swift and peaceful death. Some patients have undergone protracted deaths, at times up to four days long. Others failed to die. Thinking they would be gone within minutes, they woke up again hours later. Between the time Oregon's Death with Dignity Act was enacted in 1997 and the end of 2020, eight Oregonians who ingested the supposedly lethal drugs regained consciousness.[1] While exceedingly rare, their experiences are a painful reminder that—under current assisted dying laws—an entirely predictable death isn't yet realistic. One of these people was Louis.

For much of his life, Louis had worked as a long-haul trucker. An outdoors man, he loved traveling the vast expanses of the American West. He would sleep in the cab of his truck and go hunting and fishing between jobs. When his kidneys started to fail in his late fifties, he went on dialysis, gave up trucking, and became homeless. Louis eventually stopped dialysis. He knew he wasn't eligible for a transplant—his comorbidities and lack of housing were two firm strikes against him—and he didn't want to spend the rest of his life hooked up to a machine.

In August 2018, six months after coming off dialysis, he was admitted to a long-term care facility for Medicaid patients outside Portland. By the time Louis walked into the office of his social worker, Ada, to have his picture taken for the resident database, he was suffering from end-stage renal failure. The picture Ada took showed a man in thick glasses and a bashful smile, his shaggy brown hair slicked back in long streaks. His upper row of teeth was missing.

"He was pretty ill," Ada recalled. "He didn't hear very well, so he had to carry around a sound amplifier for you to communicate with him. Sweet man. Very gentle, good-natured person. One of the sweetest men I've ever met in my life."

Over the next few months, she and Louis became close. At thirty-two years old, Ada was taking night classes to complete her master of

social work, and she had been hired as the facility's social services director. She would visit Louis in his room, and they would sit and chat for
hours. He had recently reestablished his Christian faith, and he often
asked Ada to pray with him. He would leaf through his tattered book of
psalms, one of his last remaining possessions, until he found the passage
he was looking for. Though he had returned to his faith only a short
while ago, he had done it with the breathless zeal of someone trying to
make up for lost time.

"I think his faith was extremely important to him at the end," Ada
remembered. "He was facing the end of his life and he didn't know what
to expect. I think that he felt safe reconnecting to his faith and making
amends with God, so that he wouldn't have that burden to bear when
he died. We talked about it a lot."

During one of his care conferences with his nursing and hospice
team, Louis expressed an interest in using Oregon's assisted dying law:
he had accepted that he was not going to make it, and he wanted to
die on his own terms. Ada put him in touch with End of Life Choices
Oregon, and two of their volunteer doctors, Neil Martin and Mark
Rarick, went out to evaluate Louis in late October. His case was so
clear-cut, both physicians immediately signed off on his request. Besides
his failing kidneys, Louis had a history of respiratory problems, hyper-
tension, vascular disease, multiple neck and back surgeries, a stroke,
and a heart attack. Because of a previous opioid dependency, the pain
medications he received through hospice barely touched his symptoms.
He would lumber down the hallways bent over his cane, his skin pale
as a porcelain doll.

Louis was so close to dying, his doctors weren't sure whether he would make it through the fifteen-day waiting period imposed by the law. He barely ate anymore, constantly throwing up blood and bile. His kidneys had stopped processing waste. Over the course of a few days, his skin turned the color of faded saffron, a sign of his failing liver. But Louis pulled through, and at the end of the two weeks, Martin wrote Louis a prescription for life-ending medication.

There was just one wrinkle: Louis had no place to die. His facility forbade assisted deaths on their premises, and he didn't want to die in a motel. Louis had long been estranged from his siblings—two older brothers and a younger sister in Spokane—and the few friends he had made living on the streets were houseless just like him. Ada volunteered her apartment in the city.

"I considered Louis a friend," she said. "Here was a man in pain, and I wanted to help him in whatever way I could. So the decision was made to do it here."

It was the death of her father in 2011 that had made Ada want to become a social worker. After being sober for seven years, her father died unexpectedly of a heroin overdose, alone in his room. He had been working as a minister for the Salvation Army in a sleepy, working-class Portland suburb. She was twenty-five at the time and a nursing student, and his death changed the direction of her life.

Besides struggling with substance abuse issues, her father had been suffering from hepatitis C. Because of his depressed socio-economic status, he couldn't afford the prescription medications to treat his disease. His old coping mechanisms soon caught up with him and ultimately claimed his life. Her father's sudden death drove Ada into a profession dedicated to catching people who had slipped through the holes of a broken social safety net.

Louis reminded Ada of her father. Like her father, Louis had suffered at the hands of an economic system that prizes profit over human life, that criminalizes rather than treats addiction, and that sacrifices those who fall on hard times. Besides her, he didn't have any support in his life. And she wasn't going to let Louis die alone.

Ada knew she would be crossing ethical boundaries if she took Louis home to die in her role as an employee—but not as a friend. For the past three months, Ada had become distraught by the appalling level of care at the nursing facility. Most patients suffered from serious mental illnesses and substance abuse disorders, none of which she felt were adequately addressed. While she was there, the facility underwent a state investigation for failing to meet basic care standards. Ada had planned to leave for some time, and when Louis needed a place to die, she fast-tracked her decision. The day before his death, Ada handed in her resignation. That same day, she filled his prescription at the pharmacy.

When Oregon became the first state in America to legalize assisted dying in 1997, the law didn't specify which medications to use during an assisted death. The Oregon Health Authority didn't provide a list of approved medications either, leaving the decision up to prescribing physicians. At first, they looked in some unlikely places. They spent hours scouring pharmacological reports on animal deaths, accidental poisonings, and drug-induced suicides. Because physicians were, by law, limited to prescribing medications that could be ingested by the patient, they couldn't rely on the known efficacy of drugs that work through the bloodstream. Eventually, they settled on a handful of possible medications, knowing they would have to refine them later on.

Two medications quickly rose to the top of the field: Nembutal (pentobarbital) and Seconal (secobarbital)—both powerful and fast-acting barbiturates. At two and a half times the fatal dose, the medications put the patient to sleep, the sleep progressed to a coma, and the coma stopped the brain's drive to breathe. Between 2001 and 2018, about half of all patients in Oregon who ingested Seconal died within twenty-five minutes (twenty minutes for Nembutal).[2] But there were sporadic, unexplained outliers that took significantly longer, and five patients who took Seconal later regained consciousness. Overall, though, most practitioners thought that these medications worked reasonably well—until they moved out of reach.

Over the past decade, pharmaceutical companies have made the most effective life-ending drugs unattainable or taken them off the American market altogether. In 2011, Lundbeck, a Danish company, stopped selling Nembutal in the United States to block the drug's routine use for capital punishment. That same year, the European Union instituted a general export ban on the medication. Soon after the embargo went into effect, the price of Seconal shot through the roof. Until 2009, a lethal prescription of Seconal had cost less than $200 for one hundred capsules. Over the next few years, Marathon Pharmaceuticals hiked the price up to $1,500. Not long after that, in 2015, Valeant (a Canadian company now known as Bausch Health) acquired the rights to the medication and doubled the price to $3,000—one month after California proposed a bill to become the fifth state to legalize assisted dying.

It was around that time that physicians in Washington State started looking for more affordable alternatives. They formed a committee that included a cardiologist, a pharmacist, an anesthesiologist, and some veterinarians. Together, they set out to create their own formula for use in assisted deaths. Carol Parrot, a retired anesthesiologist from Lopez Island, said they needed the new protocol to accomplish four things: the medication had to be safe to handle, effective, affordable, and available through compounding pharmacies (pharmacies that create medications tailored to the specific needs of individual patients). The group eventually settled on a mixture of four medications by the name DDMP—an acronym based on the first letter of each of the four ingredients. DDMP contained diazepam and morphine to sedate the patient and depress their respiratory drive, and digoxin and propranolol to stop the heart. After the first thirty deaths, the group doubled the dosage to enhance its efficacy and reduce the time to death. They named the new formula DDMP2, which cost around $750.

On average, patients who took DDMP2 took much longer to die than those who could still afford to pay for Seconal. The mean time between ingestion and death using DDMP2 was over four hours in Oregon, and one recorded death lasted as long as forty-seven hours.[3] At the end of 2018, Seconal vanished from pharmacy shelves altogether (owing to a "short-term stock out," Bausch Health's website claimed), forcing prescribing physicians across the country to rely exclusively on DDMP2.

That was the medication Ada picked up for Louis from the pharmacy. It came in four separate bottles, each carefully labeled. She also bought a bottle of apple juice. Martin had told her it would help offset the bitterness of the drugs. Though DDMP2 tasted nowhere near as bad as Seconal, it was still unpleasant. All that was left for Louis to do was say his prayers and drink the lethal cocktail. Or so Ada thought.

———————

Early the next morning, a clammy, dark November day, Ada discharged Louis from the facility into her care. She drove him straight to her two-bedroom apartment in Southeast Portland. They pulled up to her building and rode the elevator to the third floor. At 9:30 a.m., Ada gave him the premedications with some apple juice.

Louis wanted to have a final smoke, so Ada walked him back downstairs. As they stood on the curb outside her building, Ada watched Louis take hasty drags from his cigarette. His eyes darted up and down the buzzing street, never lingering long enough to fixate on anything or anyone in particular. Louis told Ada how anxious he was to have God on his side for his plan. Would God receive him after taking his own life? Or would he end up in hell?

Ada could relate to the turmoil in his mind. She had been raised by a Pentecostal minister and had experienced her fair share of spiritual guilt for choosing her own path. Louis crushed his cigarette against a damp lamppost. It was starting to drizzle, so they headed back upstairs.

Around 10 a.m., Martin and a volunteer from End of Life Choices Oregon arrived. After some brief hellos, Martin went over the standard consent protocol with Louis. At forty minutes past the hour, he unscrewed the bottle of digoxin, stirred the contents into four ounces of apple juice, and handed the glass to Louis.

Martin was following a new technique pioneered by his California colleague Lonny Shavelson, who had reported success in reducing the time to death for his patients. Shavelson hypothesized that prolonged deaths had something to do with the cardiac medications in the DDMP2 compound not working as well as they should.

"The heart is an extremely resilient organ," Shavelson explained. "It doesn't stop easily, and our job is to stop it comfortably."

Shavelson began isolating the digoxin—a key ingredient in arresting a patient's heart—and giving it to patients half an hour before the rest of the DDMP2 dose. He suspected that the tiny quantity of digoxin (100 mg out of a total dose of 18,000 mg) was getting lost in a sludge in the gut before being absorbed with the rest of the medications. By separating out the digoxin and giving it a head start, he figured he would increase the speed of absorption inside the bowels. So far, Shavelson's data looked promising: the new method had decreased the mean time to death from 3.3 hours to 1.3 hours. Shavelson told his colleagues across the country about his success with D-DMP2 (the hyphen indicating that the digoxin is isolated from the rest of the dose). Like Martin, many of them adopted the new protocol for their own patients.

Louis understood that once he drank the digoxin, there was no going back. If he changed his mind and failed to take the rest of the medication, he was at risk of undergoing heart failure without being properly sedated. Reclining on Ada's L-shaped, burgundy couch, he sucked the digoxin up through a straw.

Over the next thirty minutes, Louis became more and more restless. When the time for the final dose had come, Louis was talking a mile a minute, worrying that God might not forgive him for ending his life. He asked Ada to pray with him, pausing only to swallow the rest of the medication. Still his mind kept racing.

"Do you think He's going to forgive me?" he asked Ada. "Please, God, please forgive me. Jesus, please welcome me."

Ada knew Louis to be an anxious man. The reason he didn't want to die in a motel was because he feared someone might walk in on him. She covered him with a blanket and held his hand.

"It's OK," she spoke softly. "It will feel just like going to sleep."

Louis fought the drowsiness. Like a toddler refusing to go to sleep, he grasped at just about anything to talk about. Finally, after twenty minutes, his eyelids squeezed shut and he dozed off. The volunteer glanced at her watch and scribbled down the time on her sheet: 11:47 a.m. Ada let out a breath and fell back into her chair. Louis had made it.

Over the next hour, his breathing became erratic, interrupted by long pauses—a sign that he was on his way to die. Everything looked like it was going according to plan.

***

Two hours later, nothing had changed. Not that that was unusual. Deaths on the new medication could take time. Martin had recently attended one that lasted twenty hours.

Ever since they began using DDMP2, physicians tried their best to prepare families for the eventuality of a prolonged death. But the reality always caught families by surprise. Most of them still expected their loved one to beat the odds and die quickly. In his time as a prescriber, Charles Blanke had seen firsthand how difficult protracted deaths could be on families. Waiting for someone's last breath could be very unsettling.

"The first hour or two, families are holding their loved one's hand, they get in bed with them, they don't want them to die," said Blanke. "But by hour five, by hour eighteen, they are ready for their loved one to leave this earth. And it's hard on everybody when they don't."

The search for better medications has been driven by what some physicians perceive as unacceptably long deaths. Yet there's no medical standard on how long a death is meant to last. For Shavelson, anything over two hours qualifies as a "problematic" death, anything over four as "unacceptable." But some of his colleagues disagree with the assumption that a good death must always be rapid. In a standard hospice setting where the process of dying can easily take days, an eighteen-hour death might be considered quick. And in some cultural settings, a good death is not necessarily a fast one—some dying people and their families welcome the chance for an extended goodbye.[4]

From the beginning, Shavelson insisted on being at a patient's bedside when they took the lethal medication. He asked all his patients to wear a heart and oxygen monitor when they ingested the drugs so he could watch how their bodies responded. Having these data has allowed him to differentiate—for the very first time—between a respiratory death and a cardiac death. A respiratory death usually happens within the span of an hour as a patient's system is flooded with sedatives, which send a message to the brain stem to suppress all breathing. A cardiac death lasts longer because the heart has to take up the cardiac medications to stop beating. Put simply, a patient either dies fairly quickly from the sedatives contained in D-DMP2, or they are in for a longer haul, waiting for the digoxin and propranolol to go into effect.

From what Martin could tell, Louis fell into the latter category. It had been two hours since he drank the final dose. Ada told him that she didn't mind waiting Louis's death out by herself—it could be hours, after all. Ada had seen many people die in the course of her work; she knew what to expect and what to look for. She still had her stethoscope from nursing school. Martin told her to call or text if she needed anything, and he and the volunteer took off. Ada lifted Louis's legs onto the couch—it was just long enough for him to lie flat. She slid a pillow under his head. Then she sat down at her kitchen table and pulled out her laptop. She had homework to do.

––––––––––––––––––

At four o'clock in the afternoon, Ada's ten-year-old daughter, April, returned home from her day at a friend's house. April had met Louis at a Thanksgiving party at the nursing facility, and she knew he was coming to their apartment that day to die. Ada had always talked openly to April about death—having had both sets of grandparents and her parents pass away, she didn't want April to develop any fear or sense of taboo around death. April walked up to Louis's sleeping body on the sofa, patted his head, and whispered, "Have a safe journey, Louis. We love you."

April disappeared into her bedroom. Ada asked her to stay there unless she needed anything. She promised her daughter she would take care of everything.

Watching Louis asleep on her couch, Ada noticed that his breathing was becoming more and more infrequent, typical of someone who was about to die. The color was draining from his fingertips, like an autumn leaf finally giving in to winter. His whole body had started to turn white. *He's gonna pass away soon*, Ada thought. *This is fine.*

An hour later, Louis's condition was unchanged. But Ada wasn't worried. She sent Martin a text message.

"Heart rate is slow but it isn't erratic. Respiration shallow and sporadic and temperature seems normal."

"Thanks for the update," Martin replied. "Here's my email in case the funeral home needs anything."

Ada's thoughts drifted back to the mortuary she had helped Louis pick out. Initially, he had planned to donate his body to science—he didn't have the money to pay for his own disposition. At the last moment, his sister stepped in and offered to pay for his cremation. At Ada's urging, Louis had reached out to his siblings to let them know that he would soon be gone. His sister and brothers supported Louis's wanting to be out of pain, but Ada didn't think they fully understood his reasons for wanting to hasten his death. But for a few days, it was all hands on deck for Louis. His siblings drove down from Spokane and spent one last day with him. They made his funeral arrangements, sifted through his legal documents, and picked up his remaining possessions—a few pieces of clothing. It broke Ada's heart to think about how little he had left.

Around 7:30 p.m., Louis started moving his arms, his face contorting into a grimace. For the first time that day, a bald sense of dread settled into Ada's stomach. *This can't be normal,* she thought. *Is that just the process with this medication?* She couldn't be sure.

Another hour passed. All of a sudden, Louis raised his head off the pillow and dropped it back down, his eyes closed. He cleared his throat. That was when it hit Ada. *This is bad. He's gonna wake up.* At 8:53 p.m., she texted Martin.

"He's becoming restless and moving. It's pretty difficult to watch. It's almost as if he is trying to wake up. He's coughing."

"OK," Martin replied. "I would call hospice and see if they can order some sublingual medications to continue to try to keep him heavily sedated."

Ada rang Louis's hospice nurse. Hospice patients typically have access to a "comfort pack" with sedatives, but Louis's provider had not supplied him with one. If hospice could get a sedative out to her, she could slip it under his tongue and prevent Louis from waking up, buying more time for the heart medications to kick in. Prior to taking the lethal dose, Louis had signed a form indicating that he wanted to remain sedated should he have a prolonged death or start to regain consciousness.

The hospice nurse asked to speak to Martin directly. Martin called her and reiterated his request for additional sedatives. She put him on hold to check in with her supervisor, the hospice doctor on call. Apologetic, she returned five minutes later. The doctor refused to place the order, she told Martin. As a member of a Catholic hospice agency that opposes assisted dying, he didn't participate in the law. He said he wanted nothing to do with Louis's death. But there might be a workaround, the nurse told Martin—she felt for Louis and wanted to help. If Martin was willing to sign the prescription himself, she could email it to him and send it on to the pharmacy. All Ada would have to do was administer it orally. Martin agreed.

A little after 9 p.m., he sent Ada a text.

"I'm ordering him liquid oxycodone via the hospice nurse. I'll call you soon. Pharmacy said it should take about thirty minutes."

Martin was puzzled—he had never experienced a case like this before. He started second-guessing himself. How much digoxin had actually entered Louis's body? Although he had given Louis ten times the lethal dose for a human being, the net amount was very small. Perhaps some of the digoxin had clung to the glass or even the straw? He beat himself up for not rinsing the glass and having Louis drink the residue.

Or perhaps Louis had been suffering from constipation or

gastroparesis, a condition that slows the passage of food from the stomach into the small intestine. He had been eating little and throwing up a lot. Or maybe Louis's tolerance to benzodiazepines and opioids was much higher than Martin had thought. Louis had been on oxycodone for his chronic pain and on diazepam for his anxiety. Could it be that the sedatives in D-DMP2 hadn't been strong enough to keep Louis asleep? But how could any of that matter? Louis was so frail and emaciated, he should have been gone in an instant.

It was this exact riddle that had plagued physicians since they first began prescribing life-ending medication under the law: Why was it that the sickest-looking patients sometimes had the longest deaths? After years of watching his patients die, Shavelson had a theory. Whatever illness had wreaked havoc on a patient's body as a whole had also decimated their digestive system. If that was true, then the drugs could be sitting inside a patient's dysfunctional gut for hours before being absorbed—if they were being absorbed at all.

Shavelson and his colleagues came up with a red flag checklist for these and other high-risk cases. Patients with strong hearts—those under fifty-five and extreme athletes—are on that list, as are people suffering from gastrointestinal diseases such as pancreatic cancer, those with a high tolerance to opioids and alcohol, and extremely overweight patients.

In retrospect, Louis ticked many of these boxes. But there was no going back. For now, Martin needed Louis to stay sedated so the medications could do their job.

Around 9:30 p.m., Martin received a call from the pharmacy. The pharmacist didn't have the right strength of oxycodone and needed him to approve a different formula. It would be another half hour before they could deliver the medication. Martin gave the green light, asking her to hurry.

An hour later, at 10:30 p.m., the medication still hadn't arrived at Ada's apartment. And things were coming to a head. Ada had abandoned her seat at the table and was cowering on the floor next to the couch. His eyelids shut but twitching wildly, Louis let out a muffled moan. Then he unzipped his pants and urinated on himself.

Fingers flying across her phone, Ada punched out a text to Martin.

"I'm ninety percent positive this man is going to wake up. He is aware enough to squeeze my hand when I ask him questions. He is continuously moving. This is so unnerving. He keeps lifting his head off the pillow. I honestly don't know how I'm going to sleep tonight. This was very unexpected. He's urinated on himself and actually undid his pants."

"I've just spoken with the hospice nurse who says medicine should arrive in twenty minutes," Martin responded. "I also specifically requested that the hospice doctor order medication to keep him unconscious, per his wishes."

"All right, I'm just going to stay up as long as I can and do my best to comfort him."

"That's all you can do for now."

To calm her nerves, Ada returned to her perch at the table and her homework, keeping an ear out for her door buzzer.

At 11:30 p.m., Ada saw a shadow out of the corner of her eye and looked over.

Louis was sitting up and awake. Then he vomited all over the floor.

Ada bolted to the couch and asked him to lie down. Louis stared at her in disbelief, his eyes wide with terror. He screamed, "Ada, why am I not dead? Why am I not dead?"

Her heart banging in her chest and panic sealing her throat, Ada dashed to the kitchen and yanked a pile of garbage bags out of a box and a wad of paper towels from their roll. Soaking up the fluids with one hand, she shot Martin a text with the other.

"He's awake and moving around. This is horrifying."

Her message didn't reach Martin. He had already fallen asleep.

Ada carried Louis to the bathroom—his legs were no longer working. She had noticed flecks of blood in his vomit, and as soon as the bathroom door locked behind him, she dialed up hospice. Alone and terrified, she felt desperate to not have Louis die a violent death. When the nurse on call tried to brush her off, Ada let loose.

"I don't care who brings me medication." Her voice rose in anger. "I need somebody here now to support this patient, who is in your care. He has woken up. I need medication to sedate him per his wishes. He's vomiting profusely and I'm going to call 911 if nobody gets here."

The nurse promised to be right over. Ada hung up and cracked open the door to April's room: her daughter was fast asleep; she hadn't heard a thing. For a second, Ada rested her head against the smooth doorframe. *Imagine having the courage to take a fatal drug and then waking up, realizing it didn't work,* she thought. As if on cue, sounds of retching echoed from the bathroom. Ada drew April's door shut and tiptoed toward the sound.

A little after midnight, the hospice nurse arrived at her door—empty handed. She took one look at Louis, who lay babbling and moaning on Ada's sofa. "This is bad," she blurted out and jumped on the phone with her supervisor. An hour later, Ada received permission to call 911. At 1:30 in the morning, an ambulance pulled up and transported Louis to the hospital.

The moment Louis entered the hospital, his hospice promptly discharged him. Because patients on hospice are ineligible for hospital admission, his provider could officially say that he had broken the rules. The medication never came.

————————

When Ada visited Louis later that day, she found him in the "comfort care" ward. Nurses had given him a mild tranquilizer to help with his nausea and vomiting, and they had put him in a single room to prevent him from becoming disoriented or wandering about. Louis told Ada he was glad to see her, leaning in for a hug. Louis's speech was garbled and his short-term memory spotty, but he was more lucid than she expected him to be. He still couldn't make sense of why he hadn't died. Ada didn't have an answer for him either.

Martin went to see Louis the following day. To his surprise, Louis said he still wanted to die, using the law. He asked Martin for help. The doctor felt perplexed. Was Louis mentally competent enough to make an informed decision about his death anymore? Where would he go to die now that Ada would likely not want to offer up her apartment again? Would Louis have to repeat the process of qualifying for the law? Or could he simply receive a different set of drugs on the existing prescription?

Martin promised to do some research while Louis recuperated. He reached out to state health officials and the Oregon Medical Board to find answers to his procedural questions. As it turned out, no one knew what to do in a situation like this—the law was silent on the issue, and there was no official playbook to draw upon.

In the meantime, Louis declined rapidly. Within a couple of days, he could no longer take fluids orally, and he became incomprehensible. On Wednesday, Ada called Martin to let him know that Louis was dying. Palliative care nurses had finally put him on a morphine drip.

When Ada entered his room on Thursday afternoon, Louis lay flailing in his hospital bed, pulling at the sheets, jerking his head from side to side. Ada clasped his hand. At 4:47 p.m.—five days after taking the lethal dose of medication—Louis died.

"He didn't die peacefully," said Ada. "It was a terrible death."

Since Louis's death, Ada has stepped away from medical social work. She took a job at the school district, working as a transition advocate for children exposed to trauma. When I saw her three months after Louis's death, she had just bought a new couch. Martin had offered to pay for it, but she declined. What bothered her weren't the stains; she had managed to scrub those out. It was the imprint on her mind that was harder to erase.

"I just couldn't look at it anymore," she told me. "I didn't want to sit here and have that image of him sitting up in my head."

Since 2018, Shavelson and his colleagues have further fine-tuned the drug protocol. Suspecting that the propranolol wasn't doing much, they swapped it out for amitriptyline, an antidepressant that can cause a fatal change in heart rhythm at high doses. With this change, 90 percent of Shavelson's patients have died in under two hours. Physicians in other states have adopted the new protocol, reporting similar times to death. One issue they have run into is that amitriptyline is unimaginably bitter. It can cause an intense burning in the mouth and the esophagus. Shavelson recommends a spoonful of fruit sorbet immediately after ingestion to cool down any burning. In 2020, Shavelson began adding phenobarbital as a third sedative to increase respiratory suppression, and he no longer advises separating the digoxin from the rest of the dose. The new formula, DDMAPh, has yielded an average time to death of 1.1 hours.

Despite some setbacks, the pharmacology of dying has come a long way. With increased knowledge of the risk factors that could lead to a prolonged death and with the improved drug protocol, it is unlikely that a case like Louis's would soon repeat itself.

CHAPTER 8

Family Matters

The barriers many patients face on their way to an assisted death become even more daunting without the social support to surmount them. It is usually family members—or close friends acting in that role—who serve as advocates for someone's desire to die. Kin become the ad hoc project managers of a loved one's assisted dying case: they log hours on the phone with hospice, physicians, and volunteers; help steer their loved one through the paperwork and sequence of requests; shuttle them to their doctors' appointments; procure the lethal prescription; lend moral support before and during the death; and make postmortem arrangements—all the while dealing with their own feelings of loss and regret in the face of death.

Typically, family members have been involved in a loved one's care all along, sharing in the highs and lows, so when someone expresses the desire to pursue an assisted death, their wish rarely comes out of left field. In fact, many terminally ill patients worry not just about their own suffering but about the anguish their suffering causes family members who witness their ordeals. "Relational suffering" conveys the idea that a person's suffering is never just theirs alone—suffering is always mediated by our relationship to others.

"[A person] suffers because of the pain of someone she loves—a mother, say, confronted by her wounded child," writes anthropologist Talal Asad. "That suffering is a condition of her relationship, something that includes her ability to respond sympathetically to the pain of the original sufferer."[1]

The desire to shield family members from the agony of watching their loved one die can contribute to a patient's decision to seek an assisted death, even as families willingly embrace their caregiving and witnessing tasks. Linda Jensen, a volunteer for End of Life Choices Oregon, believes that many patients opt for an assisted death in part for the sake of their family.

"That's the gift these people give to their families," she told me. "They don't hold the mental picture of a loved one in pain or gasping for air or all those things that happen when people die certain kinds of death."

Still, honoring someone's wish to die requires heavy lifting—logistically as much as emotionally—and not all families are prepared or even comfortable to offer this type of support. Some are thrown into the maelstrom of medical crisis at a moment's notice, needing to make decisions on behalf of someone they haven't known in years.

———————

In March 2018, Ruby was living out of her Toyota Prius in an Albertsons parking lot in Grants Pass, Oregon. She had been parked there for a week, reading books and sleeping, her two cats and two dogs in tow, but she couldn't remember why. In a fog, she had walked off her job as a receptionist for a veterinary hospital, loaded her animals into her car, arranged for a neighbor to look after her goats and two and a half acres of land, and started driving. For months, she had been feeling discombobulated at work, distracted by one pounding headache after another, and watching her usual capacity for empathy dwindle.

Ruby drove to the shopping center and came to a stop in the parking lot. From there, her recollections turned spotty. The last thing she remembered was dialing the number of her former boyfriend, Marcus. Her current boyfriend, Jack, was vacationing in Mexico, and she had no way of reaching him. She told Marcus that something was going on, but she didn't know what.

"My batteries are wearing down," she said.

Thinking that she meant her car battery, Marcus picked her up and took her to his house. That was when Ruby experienced a mental breakdown. She no longer knew who she was, couldn't keep any food down, and became incontinent. Marcus notified her siblings, who told him to take Ruby to the emergency room while they rushed to the hospital from hundreds of miles away. The CT scan revealed a massive glioblastoma, a malignant, aggressive brain tumor. Doctors quickly started Ruby on steroids to reduce the swelling in her brain and prepared her for surgery a week later. Her tumor had already grown tendrils like an octopus, so all surgeons could do was slice away some of its mass, knowing that any cuts would grow back almost immediately. Her surgeon finally told Ruby's family that she would never get well again. At fifty-seven years old, Ruby was looking at a life expectancy of a few months.

It became clear right away that Ruby couldn't go back home: she was at an increased risk of falling and seizures, and she could no longer move without a walker. After weighing all their options, her older sister, Beatrice, offered to take over her care. Beatrice had retired the previous year as the director of a childcare center, and she and her husband, Ralph, had a spare bedroom in their Portland home, five hours to the north. Even if their time together was going to be cut short, Beatrice was curious to discover who her sister had become as an adult and make up for some of the years they had lost. Following their mother's death, the sisters had drifted apart and hadn't spoken in more than a decade.

After Ruby joined Beatrice in Portland in early April, she enrolled in hospice care and told her sister that she would like to have the option of pursuing an assisted death. Ruby knew that Oregon had passed the Death with Dignity Act when she moved to Grants Pass from California in 2004—it had been part of her reason for moving to the state. If she ever needed to have that kind of control at the end of her life, she thought, she could exercise it. Ruby had always thought it ironic that pet owners were expected to put their animals out of their misery, while a human being in the throes of a terrible fatal illness had to keep going until the end.

Seeing how quickly Ruby was deteriorating, Beatrice decided to honor her sister's wish. She promised to help Ruby make her death as comfortable and painless as possible, no matter which path she chose. Beatrice knew it was pointless to hold out for a miracle.

"People who keep hoping that they will be the ones to beat the odds don't end up with any time to think about what is *actually* happening," she told me during my first visit with the sisters. "They get cheated out of an opportunity."

Beatrice had the self-assured, no-nonsense attitude of a primary school teacher. She kept her hair trimmed short and her house well stocked with emergency candy for Ruby.

"Who is going to tell a dying girl she can't have candy?" Beatrice joked when she showed me what the sisters called "the wall of snacks"—a kitchen shelf featuring a lineup of all the major candy and cookie brands.

In May, she helped Ruby initiate her application for an assisted death. Because Ruby didn't want Beatrice to be left with a lot of bureaucracy after she was gone, the sisters drove to a mortuary in Clackamas to arrange for Ruby's cremation (to the shock of the mortuary staff who couldn't understand why someone so young was preordering a cremation). By the end of the month, Ruby had qualified for obtaining a lethal prescription under the law. But she wasn't sure yet whether she would use it.

"My gut instinct is that this disease is going to do its thing," said Ruby, her wheat-blond hair wreathing her round face. Dexamethasone, the steroid medication she was taking, had given her chipmunk cheeks and added extra pounds to her figure. "But I want to have the option of taking the medication if suddenly things go south and I realize that I can't do this on my own. I don't want to be sitting here miserable and wishing it was all over. And I don't want to feel bad because my sister's having to work double time because it's such a nightmare."

"Well, don't worry about that." Beatrice gave a dismissive wave of her hand and reached for a glass of her handmade lemonade. Then she turned to me. "You hope that in a perfect world, hospice takes us right to the edge and that you never have to say, 'OK, this is the moment.' But if hospice is getting it wrong, we want to have the choice."

Ruby's hospice physician had told her that a brain tumor could behave unpredictably, depending on what area of the brain it pressed up against. From one day to the next, she might lose her ability to speak, become paralyzed on one side of her body, or experience sudden seizures—it was hard to anticipate. Beatrice called it the tumor's "wild card."

Even though Ruby had no idea who she would be next week or a month from now, she was clear-eyed about facing the end of her life. She knew she was all out of bargaining chips, and she accepted the inevitability of what lay before her.

"I am looking at a shortened shelf life," she told me and shrugged.

Ruby was certain that the surgery had removed parts of her brain responsible for distressing emotions like sadness or worry. Though she had never been one to wear her emotions on her sleeve, her affect had become uncharacteristically flat and detached. She could become intensely focused on certain things, but emotionally she no longer had a big range. The sisters joked about it all the time.

"We throw people off," said Ruby, "because they come in and expect us to be crying and sad."

Beatrice and Ruby spent their days around the house, reading, watching movies, and journeying to the local library. In the evenings, after dinner, they would sit around the table telling childhood stories and gossiping about the rest of their family. Beatrice noticed that her sister was increasingly living in the moment; Ruby no longer seemed preoccupied by what had happened the day before or what would happen the day after—she had grown keenly aware of her surroundings. But occasionally the gravity of their situation caught up with the sisters.

"We depressed ourselves the other day with all of this, wondering whether Ruby should tell our brother about her plans," Beatrice said. "And we both hit this low spot, and she looked at me and said, 'I should have gotten Disney movies from the library. We need to pick this up.' It was so funny. We ended up watching two movies: brainless, low, uncomplicated plots where everybody lives—even the rats. That's what we needed."

Three weeks later, during my next visit, Ruby was feeling a lot more fatigued and spent much of her day sleeping. One of her medications was thinning her skin and giving her nose bleeds several times a day. Her feet and ankles had ballooned, and she had trouble getting down the patio stairs to Beatrice's car. Ruby's boyfriend, Jack, had come up from Grants Pass to spend time with her and take her for trips in her wheelchair. He had tried to persuade her to take a final cruise with him on the Panama Canal.

"He wants to cram as much life into her as he can," Beatrice said. "It's very cute. We can only have Jack visit every two weeks."

Jack didn't yet want to think about a time when Ruby would no longer be around. It was easier to pretend that things were still normal and that all Ruby needed was a little bit of exercise or a change of scenery. Ruby had told him that she didn't expect him to be there for her death—she didn't think he would be able to handle watching her die.

"He doesn't need to have that in his memory bank at all," she said, squaring her shoulders and crossing her arms over her chest. It was the first time I had seen her express a strong stance about anything. Ruby worried about what Jack's last memory of her would be. She was thinking of asking him to stop visiting soon, while she was still in control of her body. "I'm just so aware that there's a point when I won't be here. Will I miss Jack? Yeah. But I'm not gonna be around to miss Jack. He'll be around to miss me though. He'd *better* miss me."

Ruby still hadn't made up her mind about whether she would use the medication, but she wanted to know it was going to be ready if and when she needed it. Her prescribing physician, Charles Blanke, had called her script for Seconal into the pharmacy on June 4, but she hadn't received any news since then, despite calling twice to ask for an update. She was told that they would call her once the medication was ready for pickup.

"I just don't want to be in a situation where, for whatever reason, my option was cut off from me, and I couldn't get it," Ruby said, brushing a loose strand of hair away from her face. "So right now, my main interest is 'Do you actually have a package sitting behind the counter with my name on it?' That's what I want to know."

In early July, Beatrice switched out Ruby's queen-size bed for a hospital bed, and Ruby went on a catheter. Every four hours, Beatrice dissolved Ruby's pain medication and slipped it into her mouth. During the day, Beatrice hung out in her sister's room, crocheting, reading, and playing Ruby's favorite music when she was awake. Beatrice intuited that Ruby's time was coming to an end, and she wanted to give Ruby the comfort of her presence.

In the space of a week, Ruby stopped getting out of bed, stopped reading, and spent most of her waking hours sleeping or looking out the window into the backyard. Her interest in food was gone, and by mid-July, she didn't eat at all anymore. When Beatrice and her husband, Ralph, asked her something, Ruby's answers became monosyllabic.

"It was as if you woke someone up in the middle of the night to ask a question," Ralph recalled. "They would answer you, and then they would want to go back to sleep."

As Ruby's world was becoming smaller and smaller each day, she never complained. And Beatrice never asked her sister about the status of her prescription. From the beginning, she had let Ruby handle all the logistical details of her plan for an assisted death; she wanted Ruby to be in charge and not unduly influence her decision. Then again, Ruby wasn't one to ask for help. She never rang the bell Beatrice had put in her room to sound if she was in pain—not even when Ralph and Beatrice could hear her moan in the middle of the night over the baby monitor.

"Would she ring that goddamn little bell to say come and help me?" Beatrice threw her hands up. "No."

On July 19, six weeks after Blanke had called in the prescription, Beatrice received a call from the pharmacy. The pharmacist told her that Ruby's order was now ready for pickup. He had tried to call Ruby, but her phone was switched off.

"Six weeks to get a drug for somebody who's dying of cancer?" Beatrice demanded to know. She was incredulous. Ruby had passed the point of being able to take the medication: she was in a total delirium. Her breathing had turned into what Beatrice called a "gargly death rattle," and she had stopped urinating. Beatrice sensed that her sister was actively dying.

Apologetic about the delay, the pharmacist said they had run into procurement issues. Seconal was set to expire later that year, so pharmacies didn't order the drug in advance anymore. They only kept one or two bottles on the shelf at a time.

"But it's ready now," he said. "You can come pick it up anytime."

Beatrice couldn't rein in her frustration.

"Never mind, my friend," Beatrice snapped. "She is beyond the point of being able to make that decision. She isn't even talking. We're not coming to get it."

At 3:30 the following morning, Beatrice and Ralph got up to administer Ruby's pain medications. Beatrice dissolved one of the tablets and paused. She turned off the faucet. *I'd better go check on her before I dissolve the others*, she thought.

Beatrice found Ruby dead in her bed.

A month later, Beatrice still had mixed feelings about Ruby's death. She wished she had known in advance about some of the delays in accessing the medication. Beatrice had a hard time believing that Ruby was the only person who got stumped by the system. But her grief wasn't complicated by any lingering guilt.

"I saw it as a tremendous honor to walk with her right to the edge," said Beatrice. "Was it her choice to die the way she died? I'm not sure. We have these visions of what death should be, that I should be holding your hand and saying, 'It's OK. You can go.' We can burden ourselves a lot with these things. I don't wish she were still lying here gurgling her breath. Ruby got through it without the pain and discomfort, as far as I could tell. But boy, what if she had been in pain?"

Beatrice had been talking so quickly, she had to stop for a minute to collect herself. She stared out the window where rainclouds were gathering in the afternoon sky. Ruby was gone, and Beatrice would never know if there was anything more she could have done for her sister.

––––––––––––

Though Ruby didn't have an assisted death in the end, she knew she could count on her sister for moral and emotional support. Many other families have a much harder time getting behind the idea of assisted dying. Some have religious objections to the practice, others regret that their loved one is dying earlier than they might otherwise, and some are in deep denial about their loved one's decline in the first place. When someone decides to pursue an assisted death, families suddenly find themselves face-to-face with a painful reality—the finality of life.

Robb Miller, former executive director of Compassion and Choices of Washington, has seen how powerless families can feel at the deathbed of a loved one. Throughout the eighties and nineties, he witnessed many of his friends and his long-term partner die grueling, protracted deaths from HIV/AIDS. The experience drove him to become an activist for better end-of-life care and assisted dying. Miller says he understands why some families struggle to accept their loved one's wish for an assisted death.

"Some families don't want to confront the fact that their loved one is going to die," said Miller. "And so they oppose assisted dying because it essentially rubs their noses in the fact that their loved one is dying."

Families in denial about their loved one's state might express anger at their choice and accuse them of taking the lethal medication too early, when there's seemingly more life to be lived. In an effort to put off the process of letting go, they might challenge their loved one's reasons for seeking an assisted death. Sometimes, however, those close to a patient put aside their personal objections and come together in what Miller calls "loyal opposition."

"They will remain opposed to it, but they won't interfere. That's as far as some people can get. If they are not present, their loved one might feel abandoned by them, and they might ultimately feel they abandoned their loved one in retrospect."

Those who attend an assisted death have usually decided to suspend personal grievances and rally behind their loved one, negotiating their level of involvement each step of the way. Some help a loved one put all the pieces in place but decline to mix the lethal medication or be present during the ingestion. Yet occasionally, families remain opposed to a loved one's wish to use the law and may undercut their attempt to seek an assisted death, compromising their ability to move ahead. If a dying person lacks an ally among the family, it may come down to the role of the volunteer or physician to act as a mediator.

Derianna once served as a volunteer to a ninety-four-year-old woman from Washington State who was determined to use the law against the wishes of her family. Frannie had lost her eyesight and suffered from terminal breast cancer, and Derianna remembered exactly what she looked like.

"She met me at the door every day I went to visit her, with a long strand of pearls on top of a blue satin gown, with blue eyeshadow over each eye, red lipstick on—sometimes it was outside the lines because she couldn't see—and she would hold court in her living room."

During her meetings with the family, Derianna discovered that Frannie's son and his wife, both devoted Catholics, felt distraught at the idea that Frannie would end her life and be barred from spending eternity with them in heaven. Theologically, Catholic doctrine codes an assisted death as a suicide, which could prevent a person's soul from ascending to heaven and leave it forever lost.

"The son and daughter-in-law were just beside themselves and fearful that she would be in purgatory for the rest of eternity," Derianna recalled. "But she was adamant that she wanted to go out on her own terms."

In her twenty years as a volunteer, Derianna had worked with other Catholics who didn't think their souls would be in peril because they pursued an assisted death. In her experience, even devout believers usually found a way of justifying their desire to die, convinced that a benevolent God would never want them to suffer. But because of the evident spiritual distress Frannie's decision would cause her family, Derianna started feeling uneasy about her plan.

"When her children had such a violent reaction, I couldn't support her in moving forward without first trying some other things. She needed to really consider how they would feel. And they had in their minds a truly valid and heart-wrenching fear."

Typically, Derianna would think twice about getting in between a patient's desire to die and opposition by the family. It is the patient's choice for a self-determined death that she wants to honor above all else, and volunteers don't see it as their job to dissuade patients from using the law. They are there to support someone to take this step and encourage discussion between families and patients. Derianna always talks to families about the importance of trying to uphold the dying person's wishes. She thinks it's unkind to keep a loved one from dying when they are so ill. The worst thing you can do, she told me many times, is try to hold on to somebody who is ready to die—make them eat when they don't want to eat anymore, make them get up when they just want to sleep. "That's not respect," she said.

But in Frannie's case, Derianna felt that the stakes were different. She wanted to be extra certain that Frannie had explored all other options. On Derianna's initial intake visit, she had gone over Frannie's medications with her and discovered that she wasn't taking her morphine correctly. Instead of taking it twice daily, she only took it in the morning because she couldn't read the label. At night, she had trouble sleeping because the pain kept her up. Concerned that Frannie was suffering needlessly, Derianna called her hospice nurse and asked her to review Frannie's medications with her.

Derianna also learned that Frannie didn't want to spend her money on a caregiver for herself because she intended to bequeath a large inheritance to her son, whose loss of vision prevented him from working. But Frannie was clearly well off, and Derianna knew that hiring paid help for a few months would not break her bank. She encouraged Frannie to get a caregiver to "treat her like the queen she was." Frannie continued resisting the idea, even as her son kept pleading with his mother to think of herself first.

After a few more visits, Frannie softened, and with Derianna's help, the family hired several caregivers who saw to her needs and made sure she was taking her medicine the way she needed to keep her pain-free. Once Frannie started taking the dose she should have been taking all along, her pain abated and she started feeling better. When Frannie died naturally three months later, her son was at his mother's side and sang her out.

At the funeral, he told Derianna how grateful he was that his mother was able to die in a way that would allow them to be together in the afterlife. Derianna took him in her arms. It was the only time she had worked so hard to talk someone out of using the law so the family wouldn't suffer.

"It was the right thing to do," she told me.

PART III

Regaining Control

CHAPTER 9

Flying Free

After enrolling Joe in hospice care in January 2018, Anna and Joe, the contra dancers from Vancouver, tried to qualify Joe for Washington's assisted dying law. Even with a terminal ALS diagnosis in hand, they suspected they might run into some problems with his request. Joe's physicians were all part of Providence, a Catholic health system that bars its providers from participating in the law, so they knew they would have to find their own doctors. But they weren't prepared for the level of antagonism they encountered.

Joe approached his neurologist to put his request for assisted dying into his medical chart. He wanted to get a head start on the fifteen-day waiting period required by the law because he wasn't sure how much longer he would still be able to swallow. His neurologist turned out to be even less willing to cooperate than he had anticipated. She informed him that her office couldn't help him and referred him to a palliative care specialist inside the Providence system—not to assist with his request but to discuss "alternative options."

"Everybody's choosing their words very carefully at this point," Anna recalled, a fresh swell of rage smoldering inside her. "Nobody would say there was a gag order, but it seemed like nobody was gonna talk straight with us. Everything started getting balled up, it was so confusing. Why would Joe go and see this other doctor? All it was going to do was delay his request. It felt like we were being given the runaround."

Joe quickly ran out of energy to deal with the situation, so Anna called Joe's primary care physician, who worked nearby. All she needed him to do was enter Joe's request for an assisted death into his medical record.

His response came back in an email by way of his secretary: "I do not participate in Death with Dignity." Anna called it his "prisoner of war statement."

Joe and Anna, it seemed, had reached a dead end.

"What the heck were we supposed to do?" Anna felt incredulous. "We were in a race with the clock for Joe. I just had to keep going."

Anna knew that Joe's window of opportunity was closing fast—his breathing was becoming more labored by the day, his voice barely audible anymore. Anna had to ask him to repeat a sentence several times before she understood, a sign that Joe might soon lose his ability to swallow. He could no longer go without his BiPAP machine at night. By mid-February, he was on it all day.

Joe was becoming frightened, and he wasn't used to being frightened. The drowning sensation he had been so afraid of overcame him regularly now—the feeling of being waterboarded by an invisible hand.

Samuels had told him that ALS patients produce extra saliva, which builds up in the mouth. When the saliva goes down the wrong pipe, it can feel like somebody is holding your head underwater. There were times when Joe's legs would lash out in sheer panic. And he still didn't have the medication that could put an end to his suffering in the house.

Near the end of her rope, Anna stumbled across End of Life Washington online, the volunteer organization that assists patients and families in navigating the law. She gave them a call and told them about Joe's predicament. The organization promptly sent out two volunteers to talk with Joe and Anna, and they later arranged for two of their volunteer doctors to see Joe. One of them, Carol Parrot, created a medical record in which she officially entered Joe's request. The second physician, Neil Martin, who is licensed in both Oregon and Washington, visited Joe a few days later and again after the fifteen-day waiting period was over.

Martin was the one who finally wrote the prescription for Joe's life-ending drugs. But the doctor still had to wait forty-eight hours before he could call it in to the pharmacy—another safeguard built into the law.

On February 23, 2018, Joe received word that his prescription for DDMP2 had been called in to the pharmacy. It was just a matter of days now before it would be ready for pickup. It took three to four days for the pharmacy to procure the different ingredients and compound them.

During my visit with Joe and Anna a few days later, I asked Joe if knowing that his prescription was almost ready had changed anything for him.

"It's more immediate," he said. "All the doctors have emphasized that I'd better not get too far along. If I can't swallow, I lose my chance. So that makes it very immediate."

Some patients who go through all the steps of qualifying for an assisted death never end up using the medication. They either die before they have the chance to take it or they become physically or mentally incompetent to independently ingest the lethal dose. Others have a change of heart. In the first twenty-three years since Oregon passed the Death with Dignity Act, 2,895 patients received prescriptions under the law, and 1,905 died from ingesting the fatal drugs.[1] That means that one-third of all patients who requested the medication never took it.

Joe drew in a shallow breath and glanced down at his body.

"There is relief at the idea that I'm done with it. No more of the struggling, no more struggling just to breathe, or struggling to eat. Or go to the bathroom."

I asked him how likely he thought he was to use the medication to expedite his death. Anna was curious as well.

"Joe, what do you think are the chances that this is how you're going to do it?" she asked. Raking her fingers through her heavy, silver hair, she turned her torso toward him so she could watch his reaction.

Joe paused. "Pretty high."

"Really? That's more than I thought," Anna said, her jaw tightening. She was straining to take in his words. It suddenly struck me that they hadn't had this conversation yet.

Anna kept talking. "I think you were a little, a few weeks ago, you said something like you didn't know if, when you got right down to it, you didn't know if you'd have the guts. But I guess you're getting the guts."

"Well, I don't know about that. I still worry about that."

"You're going to do it even without the guts?" Anna quipped. A nervous laugh escaped from her mouth.

"No, I worry about that part, but intellectually I'm there."

"OK." Anna forced a smile. "It's going to take guts for me too."

For the last couple of weeks, Joe had been practicing swallowing four ounces of liquid in less than two minutes whenever Anna handed him something to drink. He knew he had no margin for error. If he couldn't ingest all the medication at once, he risked falling asleep on a partial dose. If he started choking halfway through and he had to stop drinking, the drugs might not work. And he desperately needed them to work.

Anna called him an overachiever, with a fondness that instantly softened the hard edge of the term. Joe had two Ivy League degrees. Throughout his life, he had always kept extensive records of everything he did. When he still drove, he had an apparatus installed in his car that recorded his mileage and gas. Now he kept copious Excel sheets of his caregiver hours and everything else related to their joint budget. Record keeping made Joe feel secure. During their years of being partnered, his meticulousness had sometimes driven Anna up the wall. Now she was glad for it.

There were two things that Joe kept saying to Anna during his final weeks. He would look her straight in the eye and murmur, "This is the end. It's the end."

Joe had come to realize that he wouldn't live to see another summer. That he wouldn't celebrate another Christmas. That he would probably never see his children in person again. There were a lot of lasts in his life right now, each painful in its own way.

The other thing he said to Anna over and over again was "I don't want to leave you."

Joe and Anna never married—she still called herself his girlfriend—and their regret around never having tied the knot weighed heavily on them both. Joe told Anna that he had made a mistake in not marrying her. She had wanted to get married years ago, but he kept thinking they would have more time—until they didn't.

But there was one unexpected aspect to Joe's sharp decline. Knowing his days were numbered, Joe had reconnected with his three children, after not having heard from them in years. Following a messy divorce, Joe was a single parent to his youngest daughter, Denise, a high-functioning woman with Down syndrome for seven years. He later remarried someone none of his children liked. Joe suspected that his second wife said and did things to his children behind his back, but even after their divorce, he never managed to reconcile with them.

Though the lines of communication between Joe and his children had long been frozen, Anna had occasionally kept tabs on them by typing their names into search engines and tracking them on Facebook.

Joe waited until October 2017—nine months after he had sent the letter about his ALS diagnosis to all his friends—to share his news with his children.

"It's really sad all the years that were lost," Anna said. "But everybody is back in the fold now. There's a tremendous amount of outpouring of love and support."

The left corner of Joe's mouth lifted into a half smile. "The kids keep trying to figure out how to extend my life, you know, use palliative care, increase the quality of my life, but it's really not gonna work. I appreciate the sentiment though."

A full smile blossomed across his face. Joe knew his children were just hoping for a little more time. Joe had recently Skyped with Denise, who had written down a long list of things she wanted to say to her dad. He was so touched, he burst into tears.

I asked Joe if he might want to have his children there for his death.

"I don't know whether I would push my kids to fly in for a thirty-second, you know"—he was searching for the right word—"show."

Anna and I looked at each other, unsure whether we had just heard Joe make a joke. When we looked back at him, he was grinning.

"You can't stay alive for us," Anna said finally, scrubbing any lingering doubt from her voice. "You have to make the decision based on what's best for you."

Anna had told me, privately, that she had been fighting her own battle to get on board with Joe's decision. On one hand, she wanted to support his deep desire to end his suffering. On the other hand, she was terrified to lose him and couldn't imagine her life without him in it. For Anna, the most loving thing to do was also the most heart-wrenching: being willing to let Joe go in spite of herself.

As I left Joe's house and the door shut behind me, I wondered if this was the last time I would see him. For a brief moment, as I turned the key in the ignition of my car, I asked myself if I should have said anything else to him. What do you tell someone who is about to die?

On Wednesday afternoon, February 28, Anna and Joe's sister climbed into her car to pick up Joe's prescription from a pharmacy a few miles away. Joe had told Anna he wanted to have the medication in the house. Jittery and sleep deprived, Anna was glad she didn't have to drive by herself.

When the two women pulled up to the store, they found a small wooden door with the sign "Specialty Pharmacy"—a tiny storefront with a couple of chairs and an oblong counter. All the medication was compounded and stored in the back.

"I'm here on behalf of Joe," Anna heard herself say.

The two pharmacists were already expecting her. They copied her driver's license and showed her the insides of the bag: the two premedications Joe would take an hour prior to his death and the lethal drug itself, DDMP2, the compound developed by physicians in Washington State after the price of Seconal skyrocketed so suddenly. The prescription cost Anna $525—not a huge financial hardship for them, but Joe was frugal. If there was a cheaper alternative to Seconal, he was going to choose that.

Joe knew he didn't have to worry about a prolonged death on DDMP2. Samuels had told him that patients with ALS can expect to die fairly quickly after taking the fatal dose. If you can talk of a silver lining with this awful disease, Samuels had said, this was it. By the time an ALS patient takes the lethal drugs, their breathing apparatus is already so compromised that their respiration ceases almost immediately.

Anna was relieved to finally hold the medication in her hands— she had managed to fulfill Joe's last wish. But she also felt anxious: the medicine in her purse made her feel as though she was toting around a loaded gun. When they returned to the house, Anna quickly locked the drugs in Joe's medicine cabinet and went to the living room to check on him. He was hooked up to his BiPAP machine.

"We got it," Anna whispered into his ear.

Joe bobbed his head.

———————

The minute the medication was in the house, Anna noticed a shift in Joe. He was done waiting. The next morning, Joe told her that he wanted to die the next day.

Anna feared that he wasn't thinking clearly, that maybe he was having one of his panicky episodes. She reminded Joe of his mother, who had always told her son to have a stiff upper lip. Anna wanted to give his children the chance to fly in before he died. But she also sensed that he was hanging by a thread.

"You have to make sure they understand why I had to do this," Joe told her.

"Can't you wait another day for them to get here?" Anna begged him. "Please."

"I can't. I can't wait. I hope they understand."

Joe said he was absolutely sure; he wanted it all to be over. His window of opportunity for swallowing the drugs was threatening to close, and if he waited any longer, he might miss it. And then the disease would have won.

That night, Joe and Anna barely slept. Joe couldn't get comfortable, constantly needing to go to the bathroom, and he had an unquenchable thirst. He ground his heels into the mattress all night long, trying to push himself higher on the bed to relieve his back pain, which had become chronic. Joe's brother, Thomas, who was staying the night with them, helped Anna turn him over so she could massage his back.

When morning came, they all knew it was time. Joe called his children to say goodbye, and he managed to reach his best friend, who was vacationing in Hawaii.

On the morning of March 3, a Saturday, my phone rang. It was Anna. She told me that Joe died the day before. He took the medication in their bedroom, surrounded by his closest friends, his brother and sister, their spouses, and Anna.

As he lay in bed, underneath three oil portraits of him and his parents, Joe asked to have his breathing mask removed to tell one final story. Anna peeled the mask from his face.

"When I was in graduate school, right before one of our big exams,

I handed out copies of *The Lord of the Rings* to my fiercest academic rivals," Joe said. "I wanted to distract them from studying." Quiet laughter rippled through the thick intensity of the room.

"How many did you give out, Joe?" Anna cajoled him.

"Quite a few," Joe whispered, cracking his lopsided smile. His next sentence broke out of him abruptly. "Put the mask back on."

Anna said that Joe had a determined look on his face as he drew the medication up through a straw. When she heard the slurping sound from the bottom of the glass, Anna knew he had succeeded. He chased the medication with some watered-down bourbon. Everyone in the room raised a glass to toast to Joe. He closed his eyes. Within five minutes, he had fallen asleep. Forty-five minutes later, he was gone.

"It was smooth as silk," Anna said.

After Joe died, Anna spent an hour alone with his body, kneeling by the bed, studying his face, and holding him. She told me he stayed warm for a really long time.

On the phone, I could hear Anna's story being interrupted by her sobs. The line cut out a few times—I was staying at the coast, and my reception was spotty. Hovering near an upstairs window to hear her, I pressed my face against the pane.

"How are you feeling?" I asked before the connection cut out again.

"Empty and sad."

As I hung up the phone, I was reminded of something Anna told me a couple of weeks ago. She had read in an online forum for caregivers of patients with ALS that when their loved one dies, they call it "flying free"—the opposite of being imprisoned in your body.

Looking out at the waves rolling across the glittering water, unbridled and rhythmic, I wondered if Joe felt that he had been cut loose.

When illness has broken a body the way it broke Joe's, having a say over the manner and timing of your death can come as a huge relief. But not all assisted dying patients feel that they need to take the medication to experience this kind of relief. For some, just knowing they have a backup if things take a turn for the worse is enough.

Mark Rarick, a retired oncologist who volunteers for End of Life Choices Oregon, is convinced that having access to the prescription works like an insurance policy—a guarantee against the possibility of an unexpected future loss. As a prescribing physician, he has worked with lots of patients who never used the medication but who wanted to have it available just in case they decided to take it.

"That's all they are asking of us," said Rarick. "It's not about what happens—it's about the person deciding to choose the end of their life. It's not a failure if they don't take it."

Elizabeth certainly wasn't ready to use the medication anytime soon, or maybe at all. Sixty-eight years old and from coastal Oregon, she had cleared all the hurdles of qualifying for an assisted death. When I met her, she had been living with progressive cerebellar ataxia for nine years, and probably much longer. Nine years ago was when a physician was finally able to give her disease a name.

Progressive cerebellar ataxia is a rare neurological disorder that disrupts a person's balance, coordination, swallowing, and speech.

Patients with this condition often appear clumsy because they have trouble walking, lose fine motor skills, and experience painful muscle tremors. As with ALS, there is no cure.

When I visited Elizabeth and her husband, Glen, in their seaside home, Elizabeth was sitting in an armchair on the second floor, her petite frame swallowed up by the cushions. She wore large glasses, and her forearms were tinged in an almost translucent blue—bruises from a recent fall, she told me, her third that month. She had made it to the fourth step of her staircase when she suddenly tumbled backward.

"It's like someone just shoves you," she said. "It's not like you get a warning, *Oooh, I'm feeling dizzy.* It's just like BOOM. Done."

Not mincing his words, her doctor had told her that she could expect to die in one of two ways: she would either fall and crack her head open or she would get pneumonia from aspirating her food. His words rang in her head every time she tripped and every time she choked on a pea.

Elizabeth spoke in condensed bursts, like a faucet turned on and off. It made it easier for her to manage the aggravating slur in her speech. She said that mundane tasks had become a herculean struggle for her. "Just turning over in bed is a project. Something that you just do without thinking, I've gotta think and plan ahead, and I get stuck."

But what hurt her the most was having to give up owning a dog. For ten years, she had worked in an animal shelter and wrote a weekly column on how to solve behavioral problems in canines. A few years ago, she noticed she was gripping her dog's leash like a buoy on their daily strolls, trying to steady her gait. Normally, when someone's head bounces up and down as they walk, their eyes stay straight. Hers didn't.

Not wanting to burden Glen with caring for a pet on top of caring for his wife, she decided to find a new home for their dog.

Glen would have given anything to reverse Elizabeth's body's gradual loss of function. Every day, he took her for a two-hour ride in their car. They would stop at Starbucks for a coffee and head to a special spot where they could watch eagles fly. Elizabeth almost never got out of her seat, but she treasured their daily ritual. So did Glen.

"Sitting two feet away from my wife for two hours every single day, we talk about everything," he told me. "We've bonded so much more than earlier in our marriage, when I was going to work every day and she was running the house, and you talked a little over dinner and in the evening."

Every night, Glen kneaded her back to ease the pain from her falls. One night, she told him that if she couldn't get a lethal script to hasten her death, she wanted him to take a gun to her head. Glen was a retired police officer and kept guns in the house. Her request brought him to tears. He would do anything for her, but not that.

Glen recognized that his wife's wish to be done had nothing to do with him. "She loves me very much, there's no doubt in my mind about that," he told me when she was out of earshot. "But she doesn't know how much more of this she can take."

––––––––––––

During Elizabeth's next routine doctor's visit, her family physician was shocked to discover how quickly her disease had progressed in the span of a year. By then, the neuropathy pains shooting down her legs had become so severe, she would call out in distress multiple times a night.

"It feels like getting stabbed," she told him.

Elizabeth asked about her chances of qualifying for an assisted death, not really believing she would be eligible. She had heard about Brittany Maynard's case and figured that Maynard's disease, a fast-moving, aggressive brain tumor, was nothing like hers—she expected she would slowly decline until she became bedridden and went on a feeding tube. Her doctor told her that he thought she was approaching the time frame for terminality under the law but that his religion forbade him from assisting in her death. Even so, he recorded her request in his notes and offered her a brochure from End of Life Choices Oregon. With their help, Elizabeth completed all the necessary steps and managed to procure the life-ending drugs.

"If it gets bad enough, I can just be done," she told me.

My hand reached for hers as her eyes swam with tears. Her skin felt like rice paper. For the first time in so long, she said, she felt that she had a choice about something. And she knew she could change her mind anytime.

"Going this far doesn't mean I have to take it," she said.

For the moment, she still had lots of unfinished business: books she wanted to read, questions she wanted answered, lingering attachments to life she wasn't ready to give up. She was curious whether Trump would get voted out of office, eager to find out whether the Giants would do better next year. Not that she expected to live that long—her doctors had given her at most six months—but her mind clung to the idea of a future yet to unfold.

Though Elizabeth was on the fence about using the lethal drugs,

Glen witnessed palpable changes in his wife once she filled her prescription. Prior to qualifying for the law, Elizabeth had been bitter and angry about her progressive decline. Having the medicine in her back pocket allowed her to reach a new level of acceptance about her illness and the fact that she was dying. Glen watched a long-lost sense of peace and calmness return to his wife. Her meltdowns decreased and became less intense, and her humor returned. Just knowing she could take the medication if things became intolerable had settled her mind.

"The option of taking the medication is giving her back a little bit of what nature has taken from her," Glen told me. "It's like having an ace up our sleeves."

In a 2006 article for *JAMA*, the *Journal of the American Medical Association*, Christina Nicolaidis comments on the surprising effects of gaining access to a lethal prescription. After her mother's breast cancer had metastasized to her liver and bones, her mother became eligible for Oregon's assisted dying law and soon filled her prescription. What came next caught Nicolaidis off guard: her mother found a new will to live, even as her body was falling apart. She began meditating, traveled to San Francisco, and poured herself into her grandchildren. "I truly believe that having that little vial of barbiturates on her nightstand prolonged my mother's life," writes Nicolaidis. "It gave her the freedom to fight for life without the fear of a drawn-out death where she may not think clearly or be in control of her bodily functions."[2]

Going through the process of securing the life-ending medication also did something for Glen. It enabled him, as Elizabeth's husband and caregiver, to help move her in the direction she wanted to go—instead of sitting by helplessly as things turned from bad to worse.

Yet he still wasn't sure if he would be able to mix the drugs, knowing that he would be "poisoning" her, as he put it.

"I'm not going to be very happy about being the one to help you take it," he told her one night. "But if that's what you want, I will do it."

Elizabeth didn't know either if she wanted him to carry that burden. She said that she might prefer to die naturally after all. For the time being, she was content to put the issue on the back burner and return to living her life.

A couple of months later, Elizabeth caught a severe case of aspiration pneumonia—just as her physician had prophesized. Some morsels of food had slipped into her right lung and caused a bacterial infection. At first, she thought she had pulled a muscle in her rib cage and refused to go to the hospital. But Glen eventually called an ambulance. Elizabeth didn't want any treatment that went beyond comfort measures, and she had no desire to be resuscitated.

"Make me comfortable and help me die," she told her medical team, who put her on a morphine drip. By the fourth day, she was in a state of suspended animation, and Glen knew she would not come back. He took her physician aside and asked him to increase her morphine. Her physician said that his morals prohibited him from assisting someone to die.

That was when Glen lost it.

"I understand your morals, but let me tell you about my ethical duty to my wife," he spoke sharply, suppressing his urge to yell. "My ethical duty is to do what's best for her. And I don't think it's very fair for you to let your morals override my duty. She's getting really uncomfortable, and I don't want to see her uncomfortable."

For a few minutes, the physician stood stunned and stared at Glen in silence. Then he promised to dial up her drip.

Later that night, just before midnight, Elizabeth drew her last breath.

When I called Glen a few weeks after her death, he said that he missed his wife terribly. But he was trying to move on.

"When you lose your spouse, you lose part of yourself." His words resounded through the speaker. The next sound was a muffled cry. "Excuse me."

Glen told me he had recently made a donation to End of Life Choices Oregon, saying in a handwritten note that their services made a huge difference to him and Elizabeth—even though she never used the medication.

"She suffered constant pain for the last seven years," he wrote, "and she felt she had absolutely no control of any aspect of her daily living condition. You returned control to her. Thank you sincerely."

He had also disposed of the lethal medication. Following his pharmacist's advice, Glen spent four days collecting the grounds from his morning coffee and mixed the drugs into it. Then he drove out to the dunes, took a garden shovel out of his trunk, and dug a trench. As if sowing a new line of flowers for the spring, he sprinkled the black grounds into the ditch and scooped mounds of sand on top.

When he had finished, he got back behind the wheel and drove to the spot where he and Elizabeth had watched eagles soar just weeks before. He didn't expect to see any—it was already dusk and the first stars were getting tangled in the branches of the trees lining the hilltop. But standing on the barren field as the wind picked up, he felt his wife's presence.

CHAPTER 10

Crossing Over

An assisted death introduces a new element of certainty into the dying process, making the time, setting, and means of someone's death known in advance. This certainty has enabled people to cultivate a different relationship toward the end of life. Knowing when their loved one will die has allowed families to be more intentional about beginning the tasks of mourning—including forgiveness, honoring, and farewell—before the time of death, sometimes supported by ceremony and ritual.

Saying goodbye can be difficult—and sometimes impossible—when death occurs unexpectedly or even gradually. Holly Pruett, a funeral celebrant from Portland, says that bidding someone farewell while they are still alive is a cultural taboo in America.

"People think that it somehow conjures death or that you should be waiting till the last minute," she explained. "There is an idea that if you say goodbye too early, it is almost impolite somehow, to call the fact of the dying into the room sooner."

Assisted deaths break with that taboo. The ritual practices that have emerged around this new way to die invert the traditional timeline of events that occurs at the end of a person's life. Things that typically happen only *after* someone has passed away—celebrating their legacy, giving away their possessions, saying a final goodbye, and coming to terms with their death—can now start to happen *before*, with the person still present. And sometimes the very act of curating a loved one's final hours can soften the pain of their departure.

Nearly all cultures honor major life transitions—birth, marriage, death—through some form of ritual. These acts of ceremony mark a change in a person's physical or social status, signaling to those around them that an important transformation is about to take place. Rituals help give order and meaning to our messy experience as humans, setting the ordinary apart from the sacred. As an anthropologist, I have long been fascinated by life-cycle rituals—weddings, baptisms, funerals— and by the liminal space that those who undergo these transitions occupy. During a wedding ceremony, for example, a couple is suspended in an ambiguous middle state: they are no longer what they once were (two single people), but they have not yet advanced to the next stage (marriage). In many cultures, ritual experts work to resolve the ambiguity of those caught in this transitional space, shepherding them to what comes next.

In the course of my research, I came to think of volunteers like Derianna and the doctors who attend assisted deaths as ritual guides of sorts—there to both enable and ease someone's passing. They supervise the ingestion of the medications, guide the patient and family through the successive stages of dying, and declare when the transition is complete. Sometimes there are overt spiritual aspects to the work that volunteers and doctors do: they might read a farewell poem or talk to the patient and family about the importance of letting go.

Derianna had spent her whole life helping steer people through major life transitions, and she embraced the special responsibility that comes with accompanying the dying.

"I feel like I'm in the presence of glory every time I support someone that's dying," she told me. "It's part of the grace that I experience every time. I feel joy at their success, just like I felt every time I birthed a baby."

Derianna introduced me to the idea of "loving someone out," referring to all the words and actions family and friends deploy to lift someone over the threshold between life and death. She thought of herself as a transition expert, someone who helps "birth" a person to the other side. That explains why she usually said she was "doing a death" rather than just "attending" or "going to" a death. For her, helping someone die was an active and dynamic process that required deep focus and care.

The idea of dying as an active process of letting go is much more prevalent in cultures that place a large emphasis on preparing for death. For instance, among Hyolmo Buddhists in Nepal, dying is regarded as an intricate art to be learned throughout one's lifetime—a project undertaken with foresight and awareness to ensure a smooth passage into the next life and a successful rebirth. The dying cannot accomplish such a weighty project by themselves. Relatives elaborately assist the dying person in dissolving their enduring attachments to the world. They might place valued objects, such as money or jewelry, on the dying person's chest to satisfy any lingering yearnings for possessions in this world. When death approaches, those near and far gather at the deathbed so that the dying person isn't held back by their longing for their loved ones. As anthropologist Robert Desjarlais notes, "Attachment does not occur when nothing is longed for; many Hyolmo people aim for such an absence of longing when they die."[1]

Having witnessed hundreds of deaths, first as a nurse and later as a volunteer, Derianna understood the implicit dangers of unresolved attachment. During an assisted death, she always tried to impress the importance of letting go on the person who was dying. For a planned death to go well, she said, the dying person had to be ready. "They have said their goodbyes; they've done everything they need to do; they're closing that book."

She once attended the death of a ninety-four-year-old man named Melvin who couldn't wait to take the life-ending medication. He had already qualified for an assisted death months before, based on a terminal diagnosis of chronic obstructive pulmonary disease. But a recent fall had fractured his hip, quickly mutating into the axiomatic straw that broke his back. The evening before Melvin's planned death, he called Derianna and asked her to move up the time of his death. The pain from his fracture had become totally unmanageable; he could no longer use the bathroom. Already in her pajamas, Derianna told Melvin to call his hospice nurse to see if she would let him increase his recommended dose of morphine. Derianna promised to be there at 10:30 the next morning, as they had planned.

Though Derianna knew that Melvin's time was limited, she also read his urgency to die as a sign of his willingness to let go. When she arrived at his apartment the next day, she offered him her usual reminder about trying to look forward—not back—once he took the lethal dose.

Sitting on the plush carpet in front of Melvin's recliner—eye level with his pale legs that poked out of his shorts like two scrawny tree branches—she told him, "Now, I want you to do yourself a favor and do all the people who are here a favor. When you say goodbye, that's it. You're gone. You're just gonna let go and die. You put your mind to it, OK?"

Melvin held her gaze and nodded. He was a no muss, no fuss kind of guy. Originally, he had wanted to die alone, but Derianna asked him to consider his family. So Melvin had invited his son Richard to share his final moments with him.

Derianna mixed the medication, poured it into a wineglass, and gave it to Melvin, who drank it without a sound. His son Richard swooped in, gave him a hug, and told him that he loved him. Melvin closed his eyes and, within minutes, fell asleep and started snoring, his reading glasses still in hand. Ten minutes later, he drew his last breath.

Derianna believed that Melvin's death had gone smoothly not just because of the strength of the medication but also because of his ability to let go. When a person wasn't ready to let go, she said, they might take longer to die.

In the early days of the Oregon law, she attended the death of a woman whose husband was an ex-CIA agent under the first Bush presidency. While the husband helped Derianna twist open the Seconal capsules in the kitchen, he kept muttering to himself, "I cannot believe I'm doing this. I just *cannot* believe I'm doing this." The couple's son had flown in from Chicago, and he too felt uneasy about assisting in his mother's death.

Their trepidation put Derianna on notice. If the family wasn't going to support the woman's wish to die, they might cling to her and prevent her from letting go.

"Do you have anything else you have to say or do before you drink this medicine?" Derianna asked the patient as she balanced the cocktail of barbiturates in her hand.

"Not really," she replied. "I just want to make sure my family is all right."

That's a big warning sign, Derianna thought to herself. *She is not gonna die right away. She is gonna wait.*

The woman took the medication and quickly dozed off. For the next forty-five minutes, her family remained in the room, sobbing. During that time, she would stop breathing and then, all of a sudden, take a big breath and resume her breathing. The episode repeated itself three or four more times.

"I think she didn't want to die when they were crying," said Derianna. "It wasn't until everybody in the room stopped crying and started reminiscing about her life and laughing that she let go. I believe she truly wanted to make sure everybody was OK."

Intensive care unit (ICU) nurses sometimes take on a similar role in supporting a patient's family in letting go once it becomes clear that their loved one is close to death. One Canadian study on the role of ICU nurses in end-of-life decision-making notes that nurses play a critical part in helping families acknowledge and accept a patient's impending demise. The study's authors explain that ICU nurses are in a privileged place to do so—more so than physicians—because they observe first-hand the suffering that life-extending technologies like ventilators inflict on patients who are dying. Nurses, they write, help families "emotionally release their loved ones" and imagine "what the future might look like."[2]

When it comes to an assisted death, rituals can play an important role in releasing a loved one into the world beyond. They provide people with a welcome script at the end of life, when death threatens to collapse the natural order of things. Rituals offer direction and meaning to a destabilizing experience, a way to honor a dying person in the very process of letting them go.

A year before I met Jean, she had asked her primary care doctor to take her off any medications that would artificially prolong her life. After much back-and-forth, her physician relented. At eighty-eight years old, Jean was suffering from a combination of life-limiting conditions, including diabetes and a severe form of peripheral arterial disease—a narrowing of the arteries that reduces blood flow to the extremities. At this point in her life, Jean felt she was merely surviving but no longer living. By the time she submitted her request for assisted dying, her hospice physician had given her a prognosis of less than six months to live.

A week prior to Jean's first appointment with Mark Rarick, a volunteer physician from End of Life Choices Oregon, her youngest daughter, Elise, videotaped a conversation with her mother at her assisted living facility. Elise wanted to make sure that her mother had thought it all through. She knew that Jean was in the early stages of dementia, which had begun to affect her speech and her ability to retain numbers.

Elise said she took the video less for her mother's sake than for her own. When they sat down for the recording, Elise hadn't fully accepted her mother's decision. Though she respected Jean's wish to not lose control, she wasn't ready yet to let her go.

"I really wanted to understand her frame of mind and why she was choosing it," Elise told me. "I wanted to have a record, and I wanted to be able to play it back."

In the video, Jean sits in a brown leather armchair in her living room, her face illuminated by the amber light pouring out of a lampshade. A navy-blue cardigan draped over her shoulders, she cradles a bowl of strawberry shortcake in her lap. It was her favorite dessert.

Elise's voice comes in from outside the frame. "Tell me what makes you unhappy about your life right now, at eighty-eight."

"That I have no activity in my life. That I have no project that I'm working on. I miss being active," says Jean, staring straight at the camera through thick-rimmed glasses, her wispy hair tousled. She shovels a heap of whipped cream into her mouth. "The quality of life I have here is zero. I look out the window and I see these beautiful dogwood trees, but I can't see any farther than that. So this is my wall."

The camera follows Jean's glacial-blue eyes and her gesturing hand toward the grid window. Outside, the leaves of a majestic dogwood glow golden in the early evening light.

"But you feel clear that you want to end your life?" Elise presses her mother.

"Absolutely, there's no question. The only regret I have is that I won't see you grow old." Jean pauses and smiles. "But I'll watch you from above."

For a second, Elise goes silent. "So talk to me about what you see happening on the day of," she continues, her voice much softer now. "How do you see it unfold?"

"I'll have my hair done before. Maybe I'll have my earrings on. Maybe we're gonna have a glass of wine. I just…hold my hand, and I'll hold yours."

Jean had a habit of digressing and losing her train of thought. But when it came to her death, her mind was sharp. Hearing her mother be so unequivocal helped Elise come to terms with her choice. And if she was ever in doubt again, she could watch the video to remind herself of her mother's determination.

When I met Jean two weeks later, she still felt sure about her decision. All her life, she had been a mover and shaker. For seventeen years, she had worked as an interior designer in her own downtown studio. One of her proudest moments was when the mayor of Portland asked her to redesign his office. She loved entertaining guests in her home, and she loved to travel and garden. Now all the things she used to enjoy were gone. And she found herself living amid people who shared none of her passions and interests.

Thinking about her death, Jean told me, made her feel at peace with herself and the world. "I've never had any fear about dying. Every day it's getting closer, it's amazing how calm I am. And happy. Not frantic, not crying."

"The strange thing for me is knowing the day and the time," Elise chimed in, pushing her brown-rimmed glasses up the bridge of her nose. She and her older sister Valerie were sitting in on our conversation. As the director of a local nonprofit, Elise was used to working under deadlines. But she never thought she would be given a date for her mother's death.

"I've always thought death would happen unexpectedly. Even though somebody was ill, you're never gonna know exactly when it's gonna happen. With this, we're going to be with her and we're going to know. It's a sense of presence that I didn't anticipate."

Knowing the date of Jean's death had allowed Elise and her siblings to spend more time with their mother over the past few weeks; every second just felt so precious. All four siblings except one: their oldest brother, Ron.

Ron vehemently opposed Jean's decision. He had converted to Catholicism in his adult years, but his siblings suspected that that wasn't the only reason behind his dissent. Ron lived on the East Coast and hadn't visited his mother in years—he hadn't witnessed her decline the way her other children had. Elise and Valerie believed that he held an image of his mother from a long time ago, before the excruciating pain in her legs and her other health issues began.

"The two of us have done the bulk of the heavy lifting," Valerie said, her ash-blond hair parted on one side. "It's been a slow decline in several different assisted living facilities and now here. He's been completely absent from the process."

Elise nodded. "He knows that he can't prevent it," she said. "But it really irritates me that he's railing at Mom. Calling and crying. I think it's his own regret and guilt. It's upsetting her, and it's never going to change her mind."

The other day, Ron had called his mother, asking how she had the audacity to end her life. "How dare you take yourself away from us?" he barked at her. Jean hung up on him.

Elise said if Ron couldn't stand behind their mother's choice, they wouldn't invite him to her death. "We don't want him to be here if he's going to be negative. Because all energy needs to be *positive*, full of love and light, holding her as she passes."

Jean looked from one of her daughters to the other and sighed.

"There's nothing I can do about Ron," she said finally, crossing and then uncrossing her arms. "If he's going to come and cause a ruckus, I don't want him to come." She felt saddened that Ron was "incompliant" as she put it, but she was going to move forward—with or without her oldest child.

The day of Jean's death, her prescribing physician called to let me know that she would proceed with her plan. That morning, he had dropped by her apartment to make sure she was still able to articulate with absolute clarity that she wanted to die. Rarick needed to be certain that Jean's budding dementia wasn't getting in the way of her decision-making ability. Jean had answered all his questions to his satisfaction.

When Rarick, a volunteer, and I walked up to the entrance of Jean's building later that afternoon, her three daughters were milling around outside, waving and smiling when they saw us approach. Jean had sent Elise, Valerie, and Valerie's twin sister, Liz, out to the lobby to wait for us—she thought it would speed things up if someone was actively waiting. As the sisters steered us past the sign-in desk, Elise told me that, in the last couple of days, her mother had traded her wheelchair back in for her walker and her speech had cleared up.

"She's been roaring down the hallways with her walker," said Elise, her round eyes gleaming. "It's her body's last gasp."

The prospect of her death seemed to have finally put Jean's mind at ease.

Nick Gideonse, the family medicine doctor who frequently takes assisted dying cases, says that's not uncommon. Once they secure their prescription for the lethal drugs, even very sick patients frequently experience an uptick in morale and physical ability.

"The idea that once people have the prescription, they live longer, because they've been empowered, I really believe that's true. Am I a better skier because I'm wearing a helmet? No, but I'm more confident. Often, that empowerment leads to a little more eating and drinking or searching out enjoyable activities—without the fear that it will be a badly placed gamble that will leave them in a bad situation."

The minute we entered Jean's apartment, I understood what Gideonse meant. There was Jean, surrounded by bouquets of flowers, sitting in a purple armchair in violet slacks, striped purple socks, a creamy white blouse, and a peach vest. Her curly gray hair was washed and delicately coiffed, offset by silvery earrings and a big bangled necklace. Jean beamed like a school girl on the first day of class.

"Let's do this," she said in lieu of a greeting.

Jean's apartment had already been stripped down to its basics. She had insisted on purging most of her furniture, save for her bed and an assortment of chairs that stood in a half circle around her armchair. Her other son, Daniel, and Jean's friend Lloyd were sitting in two of them. Ever the pragmatist, Jean had peddled off her remaining possessions to family members and random acquaintances—whoever walked through the door, they weren't allowed to leave without something. She had persuaded Rarick to take one of her decorative African masks; I had left our first meeting with a coffee table book on Nigerian nomads.

Now, the doctor took a seat across from her. He asked her if she knew what would happen if she took the medication that sat on her kitchen counter.

"It will taste bitter, my brain will shut down my breathing, and then I will die," Jean replied, so matter-of-factly she may as well have rattled off a list of the state capitals. I was impressed. Not many patients knew the specifics of how the medication worked.

Rarick asked if she wanted to proceed.

"Absolutely." Jean flashed the doctor a coquettish smile. She had a habit of flirting with men of a certain social standing, though Rarick, looking straggly and dressed in ill-fitting hiking pants, hardly looked the part.

"Are you sure?" he probed. She seemed so upbeat, he needed to be certain.

"Yes." The first time since our arrival, the smile slid from Jean's face, and her voice turned solemn. "I want to take the medication."

Rarick handed her three pills to reduce nausea and anxiety, along with a glass of water. From my work with the doctor, I knew that each of these deaths touched him at his core. If assisting someone to die ever became easy for him, he had sworn to himself that he would quit. The bonds that he established with each of his patients ran deep.

"Thank you, dear," Jean crooned, batting her eyelashes at the doctor.

Rarick and the volunteer disappeared into Jean's bedroom to open up the capsules of Seconal. The rest of us sat down in the chairs facing Jean. Her son Daniel pulled up her favorite songs on his phone: Stevie Wonder, Peggy Lee. With one leg thrown over the other, her white tennis shoes tapping along with the music, Jean snapped her fingers and sang the lyrics she knew. When she was younger, she had played percussion and the piano.

"Is that all there is, is that all there is?" Jean and her daughter Elise belted her favorite Peggy Lee song, an anthem of Jean's mid-adult years. In the summertime, she would open all the doors in their house and, like a teenager, play the record over and over again, twirling her children around the floor until they collapsed.

Carried back to those carefree summer days, Elise glanced at her mother. She hadn't been herself in a long time. Especially over the past year, her life had turned into a reverse enactment of Groundhog Day, each day slightly more miserable than the previous. Elise knew how much she wanted out. The resolve her mother felt about her death gave Elise a sense of peace. There would be levity to her loss.

"If that's all there is, my friends," Elise picked up the chorus now, her cocked head brushing up against her mother's tresses, "then let's keep dancing."

In between songs, Jean sent me into the bedroom to check on the progress of the medication. Each time I returned with an unsatisfactory report, she raised her eyebrows as if to say, "What's taking so long?" When the powder was ready, fifteen minutes before the suggested wait time for the premedications was over, Jean's impatience got the better of her. She didn't want to wait any longer.

Her daughters scooted her armchair forward and encircled her. Their mother's urgency didn't surprise them at all. When her mind was set on something, there was no stopping her. Jean kissed each of them on the mouth. They told her that they loved her. When it was his turn, her son Daniel broke down crying. Jean tried to comfort him.

"It's all right," she said, patting his hand. "It's not all right, but it will be all right."

Welling up one by one, the siblings passed the Kleenex box between them, joking that Jean's friend Lloyd was hogging it. For the fourth time that day, Rarick asked Jean if she wanted to change her mind. She declined, so sharply I wondered if her affection for the doctor was starting to cool. He handed her the lethal dose of barbiturates. She took one sip and pulled away. Her face contorted into a grimace. "Oh, that's nasty!"

Straining, Jean forced down the rest of the drink in five big gulps. Rarick refilled the glass with water to pick up the remaining morsels of medication. He wanted to ensure that all the medication would enter her body.

Suddenly, Jean erupted into a coughing fit. Her eyes, agape, searched for the doctor's. Elise placed her hand on Jean's belly; the twins clasped their mother's shoulders. Rarick told Jean to breathe slowly. Fixating her gaze on the doctor, she took a shallow inhale, followed by a drawn-out exhale. A few seconds later, the coughing sputtered to a halt and the panicked look in Jean's eyes dissipated. The water had just gone down the wrong pipe.

Jean lit up again. "Take care of each other," she told her children, giving each a final kiss.

"Wow, that's so bitter!" her daughter Liz exclaimed, wiping her mouth. "I can't feel my lips!" The little bit of Seconal left on her mother's lips had been enough for her to taste it.

Jean turned toward me.

"This stuff tastes terrible. Someone really needs to change that. And they should change the name of the law. Death. With. Dignity. What a mouthful."

I felt a wave of anxiety pulse through me. I knew that Jean felt strongly about educating people on Oregon's assisted dying law. That was why she had invited me to her death, so I could write about it first-hand. But I couldn't believe that this precious woman, who was about to die, spent the last few moments of her life on an advocacy pitch. I suspected her daughters had expectations of some meaningful last words from their mother. Yet Jean pressed on.

"There are all these baby boomers who will want a better way to die. Our society doesn't recognize that yet. They will someday."

I promised Jean I would do my best.

Her mouth curved into a smile and she reclined in her chair. Rarick leaned in to tell Jean a story about his son, who had recently said that the country's next president should be a woman. Her eyes dimming, Jean cast him an approving look. She had long thought so herself. In the middle of his story, Jean floated off to sleep, her head sinking down to her chest.

Elise let out a primal sob. Valerie looked too stunned to cry. The sisters tried to prop their mother's head up with a pillow, but it kept dropping. Rarick recommended that Jean should lie down flat. Elise fumbled to take her mother's oversized earrings off; Valerie removed her glasses; Liz gingerly uncrossed her legs. Her son Daniel scooped up his mother from one side, while Rarick held the other. With Elise at the head and Jean's friend Lloyd holding the door, they carried Jean into the bedroom and lowered her onto her twin bed.

Jean's family stood quietly in a half circle around her bed, their hands resting on her body. Valerie distributed a call-and-response poem from a ceremony called "Going Westward to the Sunrise." It was an excerpt from Ursula Le Guin's book *Always Coming Home*. Earlier that year, the famous science fiction author had died in her home in Portland, and Elise had attended the service where the poem was first read. Jean and Ursula had been neighbors, and Elise thought that reading Ursula's poem at her mom's death would be a fitting way to usher her out.

Valerie explained that the living were to read the left side of the poem aloud in unison, pausing after each stanza so that the dying person could answer silently by reciting the lines on the right.

"We are going to help Mom cross over," Valerie declared.

Go forward. Go forward.

We are with you.

We are beside you.

Go on now, go ahead.

Leave us now.

It is time to leave us.

You are going on.

Your feet are on that road.

You are going on that

road.

Do not look back.

You are entering.

You are achieving.

You are arriving.

The light is growing.

Back here is darkness.

Look forward.

The doors of the Four

Houses are open.

Surely they are open.

I will go forward.

It is hard, it is hard.

I will go forward.

I will go forward.

It is changing.

I will go forward.

There is a way.

There is surely a way.

There is a road, there is

a way.

The singing is changing.

The light is changing.

The singing is changing.

The light is changing.

They are coming.

They are dancing, shining.

Rejoining.

The doors of the Four

Houses are open.

Surely they are open.

As our chorused voices called out to the departing soul, Elise's hands started moving in the air above her mother. Beginning at the head, her outspread fingers swept the full length of her, releasing Jean's spirit from her body. As we neared the end of the poem, her brush strokes grew heavier and longer—a kind of cleansing clearance. If death was a passage, not an ending, Elise wanted her mother to travel well.

Gradually, the color blanched from Jean's face. The intimate circle around her bed unwound, breaking away piece by piece. Rarick reached into his briefcase and retrieved his stethoscope. He pressed the cool metal circle against her blouse. It had been sixteen minutes since Jean drank the medication.

"Her heart is no more," Rarick announced, tears glistening in his eyes. Then he started crying. One by one, Jean's children and Lloyd stepped up to her body and kissed her on the forehead, whispering some final words. When it was my turn, I squeezed her arm and wished her a safe journey. Jean's skin had turned pallid already, but it remained warm to the touch.

As I watched Jean upon her bed, surrounded by her children and closest friend, I wondered what she would find in the beyond. I had once asked her what she imagined would happen to her after she died. Though Jean had attended some Unitarian Church services in her adult life, she didn't consider herself religious.

"It's a mystery," she had said, eyes trained on the dogwood tree outside her window. "I wish I knew." Just when I was about to switch off the recorder, Jean piped up again, talking more to herself than to me. "I'll run into somebody I know," she murmured. "I will look out through the clouds and watch the road go by."

CHAPTER 11

Together in Grief

Six weeks after Jean died, on a sultry summer evening, I met up with two of her daughters, Elise and Valerie, over a glass of wine at Elise's house. I was curious how the sisters had processed the experience of watching their mother die and whether they had any regrets. Had assisting in their mother's death allayed their feelings of loss and grief—or magnified them?

The day of Jean's death, after the doctor and I left, someone called the hospice nurse who had been waiting in the lobby. Jean hadn't wanted her there for her death, so they had agreed that she would come in later to pronounce her death and call the mortuary. Everyone else trickled out until only the hospice nurse and the three sisters remained. They spent two hours waiting for the mortuary staff to arrive. Elise and Valerie were surprised by how grateful they felt for the extra time. They kept wandering into the bedroom to take in the image of their deceased mother.

"Being able to be with her body felt really sacred to me," Elise recalled, sitting cross-legged on her sofa next to her sister and cradling a glass of red wine in her lap. "I kept going in the other room and looking. And I touched her. It was like a wave just really sinking in that she was gone. It felt like her energy had left her body and I thought, *That's not my mom.*"

"Yeah." Valerie nodded. "I thought, *OK, Mom is in the next room.* But I didn't think of her as Mom—I didn't think of her as anybody. It felt like something had left the building."

Elise and Valerie felt pleased with how the mortuary staff handled what came next. They showed up with a gurney draped with a quilt, gently lifted Jean's body onto it, and placed a rose on her pillow. Then they made the bed. The three sisters walked their mother's body out, helped load her onto the vehicle, and watched the van drive away.

The morning after Jean's death, her children gathered to tidy up her apartment and clear out the remaining furniture. Then they all dispersed. It was only a day later that the reality of their mother's absence set in: Elise and Valerie were knocked over by a flood of grief.

"It's one thing to say, 'Yes, that's what she wanted,' and 'Yes, she's not suffering anymore,'" Valerie said, her lips trembling. She pulled a tissue out of a box and balled it up in her hand. "But then, I missed her so much. And I still do. Losing your mother is so primal. But it helps to know she died the way she did. I think it would have been much more difficult if she had passed and was by herself."

"It felt so complete that we were there," said Elise.

"So not alone," Valerie agreed.

"And it was so great." Elise's face brightened. "It was very sweet."

Even when the time and place of someone's death are expected, death itself can come as a shock to those left behind. Still, an assisted death carries a degree of certainty that a home death on hospice does not. By the Bay Health, a hospice organization in Northern California, conducted a three-year-long study comparing experiences of grief in medically assisted deaths to traditional deaths on hospice.[1] They found that survivors of assisted dying patients reported having less unfinished business and a much greater sense of control over the dying process than those who witnessed an unassisted hospice death. Instances of complicated grief after an assisted death occurred in only two instances: when a family member remained opposed to their loved one's decision until the end or when a loved one planned to take the lethal medication but died before being able to do so. In the latter case, survivors suffered regret from their perceived failure to give their loved one the death they desired.

Readying themselves for their mother's death gave Elise and Valerie the opportunity to decide how they wanted to leave things with her. Though the sisters had different fathers and weren't anything alike in appearance or temperament—Valerie lean, petite, and a little reserved; Elise curvy, tall, and gregarious—they were the closest among the siblings, much closer than Valerie was with her twin sister, Liz. When they were younger, Valerie, at age twelve, helped to raise Elise after their mother tried to devolve herself of the burden of bringing up a fifth child. It took Elise years to work through her feelings of being abandoned by her mother.

In the time leading up to her mother's death, Elise reassessed and ultimately reframed their relationship, deciding that she could forgive her. Elise said she felt very complete with her mother at the end.

"I didn't feel a lot of anger toward her anymore," she said. "I felt a lot of love, and I just really wanted an assisted death for her because she was so miserable, and she was not living a life she had ever lived. So there was a lightness to the loss."

My mind flashed back to the glimpse of affection between Elise and her mother when they had sung along together to Peggy Lee minutes before Jean drank the medication. Now that fleeting moment of tenderness between mother and daughter felt even more salient.

Valerie chimed in. "I felt that too. She wasn't always an easy person to be with; she didn't always act very motherly. But during the period leading up to that day and certainly on that day, I made a conscious decision to let go of all that. And knowing that her death was coming allowed me to start grieving early. Instead of not being able to say something at the end and regret it later, I was able to say everything."

Elise pulled out her phone and scrolled through the pictures. She handed it to me. "The picture you took fifteen minutes before she passed says it all."

The afternoon of Jean's death, the family had posed for a final photograph. The picture shows Jean dressed up and seated in her purple armchair, circled by her children and best friend, everyone radiating contented harmony. You might have thought it was her birthday.

Elise said that Jean looked like her mother from twenty years ago.

"She was so full of life and clear, happy."

Families who think they have more time before someone dies

sometimes don't do the difficult work of reconciliation. Even on hospice, it's not always possible to be sure when the end is near. When a death is assisted, there's no denying what is about to happen. And while not everything can be solved at the end of someone's life, knowing when a loved one will die brings the chance to try to right past wrongs—to forgive and to be forgiven.

Despite the fact that many families find comfort and empowerment in assisting in their loved one's death, they sometimes face a difficult period of bereavement socially. The societal stigma that continues to cling to the idea of ending your own life can prevent families from sharing the details of how their loved one died. Many families fear being judged by relatives, friends, or colleagues for allowing their person to go through with their decision. Bereavement experts refer to this type of mourning as "disenfranchised grief"—hidden grief that is not fully acknowledged or even allowed by society. Disenfranchised grief describes the feeling that a loved one's death—such as from a suicide, a drug overdose, or a miscarriage—is not seen as worthy of the same grief as other deaths, causing survivors to keep their pain bottled up.

Sometimes the criticism survivors absorb from outsiders is subtle. It lives in the silences of things someone doesn't say, in people's offhand gestures or remarks, a body recoiling, the intonation of a word. Elise had expected one of her fellow board members to be supportive when she confided in him about her mother's death. His reaction unsettled her.

"My *God*, I am *so* sorry," he exclaimed, as if witnessing her mother die had been horrific and traumatizing. Valerie's supervisor at work emitted a hushed groan when she disclosed how her mother had died, offering no condolences for her loss.

"After that encounter, I only revealed the details to trusted friends and family," Valerie said now, her mouth setting into a hard line. "It added a layer of sadness to expend energy trying to figure out what someone's reaction might be. The experience of Mom's death was so overwhelming that to just say 'my mom died' didn't begin to express how I was feeling."

The judgment didn't just come from people outside their family circle. Valerie said she felt shamed by her own family for supporting her mother's wish to die—especially Jean's twin sister, who called Valerie after her death to say that she "felt sorry" that Jean had to "do *that*." Valerie responded that she didn't feel sorry at all; put in her mother's position, she would have done the exact same thing. Her aunt didn't say much after that.

"I will defend Mom's decision to the day I die," said Valerie, searching for Elise's eyes. Elise reached for her hand.

———————

The ability to time and anticipate someone's death can allow family members to mend bridges and reach closure with a loved one before they die—opportunities often unavailable to those who die at the mercy of chance, an unexpected medical event, or a sudden accident. Robb Miller, the right-to-die activist from Seattle, says that most families who go through the process of an assisted death are much more prepared for their loved one to die than those who do not. For Miller, an important part of that preparation has to do with all the steps a patient needs to take to qualify for their state's assisted dying law.

"People who are using the law have acknowledged that they're dying. Family members may still be in denial about it, but the very fact that the person has pursued the law and acquired life-ending medication is a strong indicator that death is coming. And that acknowledgment of death coming helps people prepare for the death—both the dying person and their survivors. I think that preparation—that acknowledgment— that life is coming to an end is an essential step in what I would call a good dying process. And it often leads to less complicated grief. There's a certain purposefulness to the dying that results in survivors feeling better about the death."

Linda Ganzini, a psychiatrist at the Oregon Health and Science University, has studied the effects of assisted dying on survivors, and she largely agrees with Miller's take. She notes that families of Oregonians who requested an assisted death felt much more prepared for their loved one's death than those who didn't go through this process. They also felt more accepting of the fact that their loved one had died: over 90 percent reported being satisfied with their opportunities to say goodbye.[2]

Ken's oldest son, Zack, took comfort in knowing that his father got to die on his own terms. Zack lost both of his parents in quick succession—one by an assisted death and one not. A week after Ken's death, his wife, Clara, slipped late at night on her way back from the bathroom. She fell and hit her head on the corner of the doorjamb. Zack's brother, Tony, met her in the emergency room and sat with her until four o'clock in the morning. The brothers hadn't told their mother yet that Ken had died; they had wanted to tell her together. When Zack and Tony saw her a day later, they told her that Ken was gone and that he loved her, unsure she would hear or understand them but wanting her to know anyway. She fell asleep and didn't wake back up. Two days later, Clara died.

When we spoke three months later, I asked Zack how the manner of his parents' deaths had affected his grieving: was his father's planned death more or less difficult than his mother's accidental death after her fall?

Zack said the fact that his parents' deaths occurred so close to each other was much harder on him than the way they died.

"After my mom passed, I cried on my wife's shoulder for hours because I suddenly was an orphan," Zack told me. "But the circumstances of Dad's death made it easier for me to accept his passing. I think knowing that my dad was going to go gave us the opportunity to say all the things we needed to say. So it helped with the grieving process in that sense."

Anticipating his father's death had tempered Zack's feelings of loss, making the process of grieving slightly less painful. Since his father's death, Zack had built a new woodshop at his house, and it saddened him that he wasn't able to share it with the man who taught him how to work and build things with his hands. He missed Ken's mentorship and advice.

"I'm having trouble with my fourteen-year-old daughter, and my first response is to pick up the phone to call my dad. And that's no longer there. There's an emptiness there."

A month prior, the alarm on his phone had rung to remind him of his mother's birthday, and for a split second, Zack thought he needed to call Ken to remind him. When reality hit, a surge of melancholy rolled over him. More than anything, it was Ken's abrupt absence that pained him. His dad's departure had left a big hole in his life.

"We miss him very much, which is something I would have been saying soon regardless of his choice," he said finally. Even if Ken hadn't expedited his death, he wouldn't have lived much longer. His health had been failing him for a long time.

Unlike the expected loss of his father, Zack experienced the loss of his mother in stages. Alzheimer's had ravaged Clara's mind for years, and for the last two, she hadn't recognized him as her son. The death of herself had preceded her physical passing. Zack had already mourned losing his mother for who she was some time ago.

"My mom had been gone for so long on a mental level that I already went through a grieving process with her. She was a shell of a person to go visit. There was nothing left of the woman that had raised me. But when she died, I still felt like I lost her a second time."

Zack and his younger brother, Tony, planned to spread both of their parents' ashes together in the forested city park that Ken had picked out for his remains. A year later, Zack continued to feel at peace with his dad's decision. He expressed a sense of solace that Ken was able to have the death he wanted.

"I still feel that Dad's choice was the correct one," Zack wrote in an email, "and I am very thankful that you, Dr. Martin, and Derianna were there with us."

How survivors grieve depends not just on the manner of their loved one's passing but on the circumstances and feelings that preceded their death.

"Grief is singular, bound to those who suffer from it," writes anthropologist Robert Desjarlais. "Grief itself cannot be shared, much as a wound cannot be shared. That cut is a person's burden alone."[3]

Regardless of how someone dies and whether they are able to choose the time of their passing, any death has the potential of feeling terribly ill-timed for those who remain behind. That is what happened to Joe's partner, Anna.

A week after Joe's death, Anna invited me back to their house. As I wound my way through their hilltop neighborhood, the rain crashed against my windshield just as it had the day I first met Joe. Right when I signaled to pull into the driveway, the garage door popped open, and Anna's car, coming from the opposite direction, lurched in. Amused by our impeccable timing, I flashed Anna a smile as I turned off my engine. But she stared blankly ahead and motioned for me to follow her into the house.

Inside it was dark and cool. Even after we entered the house, Anna kept the lights turned off. I noticed that she wore the same plaid shirt she did the first time I met her. But she looked older today and worn out, the rings under her eyes so deep I wondered if she had slept at all.

"I feel so lost," she said, dropping her grocery bags down on the counter. "I just keep wandering around the house, expecting him to be there."

Today was the first time she had been out of the house since Joe's death six days ago. She had been subsisting on peanut butter and jelly sandwiches and *Law and Order* episodes. Joe's healthcare providers had stopped by to pick up his hospital bed and some of his medical equipment, and Anna had gotten rid of his electric toothbrush and shaver to make room in the bathroom. But she had hung on to all his other belongings, her way of still feeling his presence. As we talked, she got up and changed into one of Joe's shirts—a checkered blue button-up that made her look even more forlorn. If we think of life as a continuous process of forging attachments, then death demands the careful unmaking of all these linkages.

"It breaks my heart that I won't get to see his face again," Anna told me as we stood in her kitchen, her eyes filling with tears. Adding to her grief was the difficulty she was having remembering Joe before his diagnosis—the shadow of the last year and a half a thick curtain that obscured her view. The last few years had been so intense, they had obliterated her memories of happier times.

Members of the contra dance community had reached out to her, offering their help in organizing Joe's memorial service. Anna was grateful for the help, but she kept them at arm's length. She didn't think she would get back into dancing again—the association with Joe was too painful. For Anna, there was no foresight and planning in the world that could have equipped her for the shattering blow of Joe's absence.

Anthropologists who study grief have observed that people who mourn the death of a loved one frequently "become" dead themselves, if only for a while. In processing their loss, mourners seek to become one with the deceased. Among Merina in Madagascar, for example, mourning entails "an attack on oneself," write Maurice Bloch and Jonathan Parry.[4] Female mourners deliberately make themselves look unattractive to resemble their deceased kin: they stop plaiting their hair, wear tattered clothes, and sit on piles of dung while receiving condolence visits. Right before the burial, they throw themselves on the corpse as a manifestation of their desire to join their loved one in death. These expressions of grief last until the conclusion of the last funeral rites, when mourners are reintegrated into society and resume their regular roles.

Joe's memorial service took place at one of Portland's oldest dancing venues on a balmy evening in April. Anna wanted me to come to say a few things about my work with Joe and meet some of the people in his life. She told me she was doing better.

"The more time goes by, the more I think of him as standing up tall, dancing with me, being my guy instead of my patient." She let out a shy chuckle.

By the time I walked into the dancing hall, the ballroom floor was swarming with guests. Everyone wore a name tag that featured a short note of how they knew Joe. "Dancing," I read over and over. On a table in the back, Anna had spread out Joe's running medals and bibs, along with his signature dancing outfit: a tuxedo T-shirt, black dancing shoes, and an elegant black hat. One of Joe's friends had built a diorama dance stage from wood and placed a small figurine of Joe in the center of it, surrounded by a circle of dancers.

The message of the service was consistent: Joe was a beloved friend and a competitive dancer—quiet, humble, funny, gracious, and sharp witted. After words from Joe's family and some of my recollections of him, a string of dancers climbed the stage to the sound of "Amazing Grace" on bagpipes, Joe's favorite instrument.

"He probably dances eight nights a week now," one of them said.

"Dancing with Joe was pure logical, analytic joy," offered another.

Laughter rang through the hall.

"We lost one of our best leads," a third woman said, wiping a tear from her cheek.

Toward the end of the service, a male dancer took the stage.

"Death feels like the middle of the song," he said and started in on a ballad, his voice smooth and sonorous. Halfway through the song, he stopped. For a second, he paused, letting the effect sink in. Silence hung like a ripe pear waiting to drop.

"Joe was always first to arrive, last to leave," the dancer carried on. "Except this time. He left too early."

Before the service, hardly anybody knew that Joe had hastened his death. His life had been cut short by a devastating disease, and many of his friends figured that his progression with ALS had been especially swift. That Joe had shaved off a few months of his life by taking a lethal dose of medication, what difference did it make? Joe's death felt out of sequence—even if it had come later, it would have felt too early.

PART IV

The Way Forward

CHAPTER 12

New Frontiers

I first met Bruce on the marble steps of the Oregon State Capitol in February 2018. Despite being legally blind, the grassroots activist had driven 120 miles from coastal Florence to Salem for a fifteen-minute meeting with Caddy McKeown, the Democratic House Representative for his district. Bruce was here to persuade McKeown to support a new bill that would expand access to Oregon's Death with Dignity Act. He felt frustrated that the law excluded folks like him who were suffering from a progressive, neurodegenerative disease that wasn't imminently fatal.

Bruce was diagnosed with Parkinson's in 2011, at the age of fifty-eight. His diagnosis forced him to retire early from his job as an engineering technician in the Sacramento valley and go on disability. Because the valley heat aggravated his symptoms, Bruce and his wife, Kathy, soon decided to migrate to a cooler climate. They landed in a small town on the Oregon coast known for its magnificent dunes and old growth forests, purchased a house on a third of an acre, and acquired five dogs. Over the next few years, Kathy watched her husband blossom and rediscover his appetite for life.

"One thing people don't know about Parkinson's is that it often goes hand in hand with depression and anxiety," Kathy told me. "Shortly after his diagnosis, he went on medications for depression and anxiety, and he was not very healthy. When we came up here, he said, 'I'm going to get better.' And, of course, that doesn't happen with Parkinson's, right? Well, by golly, he did. He got better."

Bruce made friends with other outdoor enthusiasts with disabilities and ventured on hikes and fishing trips with them. He even bought his own fishing boat. One of the pictures Kathy took shows him holding two giant rainbow trout by their mouths. Below his weathered, bulbous nose, Bruce sports his best lizard smile.

But Bruce also knew his late-life honeymoon wouldn't last forever. And he wanted a say in how things were going to end for him. He had picked Oregon in part because he had heard about the state's assisted dying law; he figured he would like to use it if his suffering became unbearable. What he didn't realize at the time was that the law was reserved for people with a terminal illness and a life expectancy of six months or less. However debilitating, his open-ended diagnosis made him ineligible.

Bruce's gradual loss of physical function wasn't his biggest concern: he feared that his mind would go before his body. He was already suffering from memory loss. Bruce was afraid of what might await a husky guy like him—six feet tall, 260 pounds, a former football player—in a memory care facility, where unmanageable patients are sometimes sedated and tied down. While visiting a friend's sister in one such facility, he had seen patients wearing each other's clothes and wedding bands and sleeping in each other's beds. His friend's sister, who had advanced dementia, would do wall "art" with her excrement. During his visit, Bruce had learned the term "sundowners"—patients who become disoriented and confused after dusk. "When the sun goes down, you go down with it," a nurse had said.

"I'm *not* gonna suffer," Bruce told me during our first phone talk. "I want to be able to take advantage of our Death with Dignity law."

Yet not in its current form. Bruce knew that no doctor would give him a six-month prognosis based on Parkinson's, and he was concerned that even if he did eventually get one, he might no longer be of sound mind or have lost the ability to self-administer the medication. The law's time frame for terminality would have to change.

In 2017, Bruce sprang into action. He churned out letters to the editor of his local paper. He joined Toastmasters to sharpen his public speaking skills. He sold his Babe Ruth autograph and used the money to launch a state-wide advocacy tour to retirement homes, veterans' groups, community centers, churches, radio stations, and lawmaker offices. He crashed public hearings on related bills to drum up support for his cause. During one hearing on a new advance directive, Bruce spontaneously rose to speak. "We're tired of seeing people that are lying in bed for ten to twelve years that really don't want to be there," he thundered off the cuff, "and the doctor won't tell them they have six months to live."

Bruce had never been very political. He had no experience lobbying or campaigning, he wasn't polished or even strategic, and he would often blurt out the first thing that entered his mind. Kathy lovingly called him a "loose cannon." With her help behind the scenes, he cobbled together a website for his new nonprofit, End Choices. He had T-shirts made with the slogan "My Life. My Death. My Way." But what he lacked in finesse he made up for in charm and a scrappy attitude. Bruce knew how to talk to people. He could talk to just about anyone who was willing to listen. He had managed to get Derek Humphry, the famous right-to-die activist, to be on his board of directors. And he snuck his way onto the calendars of busy legislators, like Caddy McKeown, to secure sponsors for amending the law.

As Bruce and I made our way past clusters of polyester suits to Caddy McKeown's office, Bruce gripped the handle of his cane until his knuckles showed. He still got nervous every time he pitched his ideas. There was a lot on the line for him. When we took a seat across from McKeown, Bruce cut right to the chase.

"The law's too restrictive, and we need to make it more compassionate," he said, his voice shaky and dry. He scooted a sheet of paper with the proposed bill across her desk, apologizing for the tremor in his hand. "Sorry, Parkinson's is making me get ahead of myself. All we're asking is that people have a fair choice when they know their end of life is coming."

McKeown made a steeple with her fingers and leaned back in her chair. She said she had a friend with ALS and another friend with a slowly progressing genetic disease who had lost use of his hands. She asked Bruce if changes to the bill could be legislated or if they would have to go on a ballot.

"We can legislate it," Bruce declared, his natural confidence restored.

"I'm in favor of this," McKeown said finally. "Knowing you have control is very important." But she said she worried about how changes to the law would be received in rural areas, home to her more conservative constituents.

Bruce latched on to the in-favor part.

"So can I use your name?" he forged ahead. "Your word is good enough."

"Possibly. Let me think about it."

And our time was up. McKeown's assistant photocopied the proposal and ushered us out into the hallway. As we rode the elevator to the lobby, Bruce told me he was happy with how it went. He had made a personal connection.

"Baby boomers all know people who are sick," he told me and smiled. His challenge was to translate that shared fact into political will.

A year later, Bruce had found a handful of lawmakers who were willing to sponsor an expansion of the law. For the 2019 legislative session, four separate bills entered the House and Senate floors, proposing several amendments to Oregon's Death with Dignity Act. Bruce was involved in two of them. The most ambitious of these bills (House Bill 2232) aimed to expand the definition of a terminal disease to "a disease that will, within reasonable medical judgment, produce or substantially contribute to a patient's death."[1] In other words, a seriously ill patient would no longer have to have a six-month prognosis to qualify for the law. The proposal also broadened the definition for self-administration, which would include other methods of delivery besides ingestion (opening a pathway for intravenous medication, as long as the patient was able to administer the drugs themselves).

Opposition to the amendments came from all the expected quarters—Oregon Right to Life, the Catholic Church, and Physicians for Compassionate Care—and some unexpected ones. Compassion and Choices and the Death with Dignity National Center, the two biggest national right-to-die advocacy groups, resolutely opposed the bills. Fearful of losing the ground they had so carefully carved out over the past two decades, both groups argued against any expansion of the law. One of their executives told me that until at least half of all states had passed an assisted dying law, they would not support any changes to the bedrock Oregon model. Such interference would only feed into the "slippery slope" arguments of opponents, jeopardizing legalization in future states. Prudence was the name of the game. Bruce called it "not rocking the boat."

When the 2019 session concluded, only one amendment to the original bill had made it through, with Caddy McKeown's support. Patients who were judged to be within days of their death could request to have the fifteen-day waiting period between their first and second oral request waived, and a physician no longer had to wait forty-eight hours after the written request to order the medication.

Bruce was disappointed. But he vowed to be back for the next session in 2021.

Besides Oregon, a handful of other states have witnessed efforts by private citizens, physicians, and lawmakers to augment access to assisted dying and make these laws more inclusive. The most common proposed amendments have been modest: to shorten or waive the waiting period and to expand the prescribing and consulting roles from physicians to other clinicians. In 2021, New Mexico became the first state to pass an assisted dying law that deviates noticeably from the traditional Oregon model, making it the most accessible law in America. The law contains no two-week waiting period, and nurse practitioners and physician assistants can be prescribing providers, as long as the second provider is a physician. If a patient is already enrolled in hospice, they need only one provider to sign off on their request.

What remains to be done to improve the options for patients who want some control over the end of their life? Passing assisted dying legislation in all fifty states would be a first step. As of this writing, 80 percent of Americans live in a state without legal access to assisted dying. When faced with unmitigated suffering at the end of their life, people in these states have to resort to covert (and potentially dangerous) DIY methods to hasten their death, voluntarily stop eating and drinking, or travel to Switzerland to die. We need to do better for those who are sick now and those who will be sick soon.

Moving assisted dying out of the shadows and into the public eye could be a vital second step. One way to do that is to stop referring to assisted dying as "suicide" and recognize it as a medical act. An assisted death sits in a moral and legal category of its own, and it is time for our shared language to reflect that. Here are other possible actions: make end-of-life care an integral part of medical school training, train interested clinicians in how to respond to assisted dying requests, and introduce a universal referral clause for providers who object to the practice.

Another step is to enhance cooperation with hospice and palliative care providers whose training and expertise in caring for the dying could be a critical asset. Some progress has already been made. There are hospice physicians who serve as consulting physicians on assisted dying cases, and some hospices in California, Oregon, and Washington have developed clear policies to support patients who seek an assisted death.

Lonny Shavelson, the Berkeley physician who helped pioneer the science of dying, thinks that assisted dying should ultimately become an acceptable part of hospice care, as one more option at the end of life.

"I really want assisted dying to become part of hospice protocol," Shavelson explained. "Hospice doctors have all the experience you need in aiding a death. Hospices have the capacity to make house calls, and they have experience with death and all the alternatives to an assisted death you can imagine. They know how to be at deaths. They know what deaths are about, and this is just one more form of dying. I really think that assisted dying should be in the realm of people who do dying all the time."

When he ran his own assisted dying practice, Shavelson closely collaborated with the two biggest hospice providers in the Bay area, who called on him as a prescribing physician while they acted as consultants. Their nurses regularly attended assisted deaths. Shavelson says the next step is to encourage hospice physicians to be comfortable serving as prescribers.

As new states are rolling out assisted dying laws, a new cohort of physicians will be joining efforts to tackle the science of dying, building on a rapidly growing body of knowledge. One step to improving the science of dying requires better and more standardized data collection. Matthew Wynia, a bioethicist at the University of Colorado, says that formalizing assisted dying research and data sharing is imperative to advancing the field. He now helps lead the research wing of the American Clinicians Academy on Medical Aid in Dying, a nonprofit founded in 2020 that serves as a national resource portal for clinicians and patients. As part of these efforts, the question of backup medications will need to be addressed—medications that can be safely administered if a patient experiences a protracted or difficult death.

Meanwhile, some gray areas in assisted dying laws should be clarified by legislators, especially regarding the aftermath of unsuccessful deaths and disposing of unused medications. As of now, physicians, pharmacists, and state health officials are forced to make up the rules as they go. Assisted dying laws could also be made more inclusive and less onerous to access for patients with prolonged, incurable diseases like ALS. This could be done by broadening the scope of terminality for neurodegenerative diseases, expanding methods for administering the medication, and ensuring that all patients have access to providers who will fairly evaluate their request. Patients whose insurance won't cover life-ending medication and clinical appointments should be eligible for financial assistance to defray these costs.

Other questions raised by assisted dying laws won't be resolved easily. One of these is the thorny issue of what to do for patients suffering from advanced dementia, who can't use assisted dying laws because of their inability to make informed decisions. Over the next forty years, the number of Americans living with Alzheimer's, the most common form of dementia, is projected to more than double.[2] And some of them might prefer not to live out the full course of their illness. There are theoretical discussions underway about putting in place advance care directives for patients in the early stages of dementia, which would detail their desire to die at a certain point in the future when their disease has progressed past a certain threshold. Such directives might list particular conditions that would trigger an assisted death, like when a patient no longer recognizes their loved ones, when they are unable to feed themselves, or when they become bedbound.

It seems unlikely that these proposals would gain widespread popular support. If a patient with dementia is unable to confirm their request to die when the point of incapacitation is reached, what physician is going to hold their feet to the fire and force them to die? Physicians continue to see their duty to the patient's *current* self as primary, not to their past or future self. What if the patient had a change of heart but is unable to communicate it? What if they *do* still find joy in their everyday existence, despite their wish years ago to hasten their death when they could no longer recognize their grandchildren? An assisted death hinges fundamentally on the idea of voluntary self-determination; in order to express that volition, a person must be capable of giving consent in the here and now.

Though we may never have an acceptable solution for patients with dementia, one possible avenue would be to expand the scope of terminality for assisted dying and allow patients suffering from early-stage dementia to hasten their death while they are still in control of their mental faculties, as is possible under Canada's assisted dying law. Yet taking that route would mean substantially shortening one's life span to avoid a dreaded future—something few people might be willing to do.

The ultimate challenge to address is our society's enduring denial of death. Because if death has become the enemy, we will always lose the war. When people try to sidestep their mortality, facing its inevitability becomes incredibly painful. To break through the silence and avoidance that shape American attitudes toward death, we must teach people, young and old, different ways to engage with the end of life. Rather than shield them from the specter of mortality, we need to give them the space and tools to explore their own relationship to it. By initiating conversations about the end of life early on, we might regain our lost societal knowledge of death. And a deeper awareness of our impermanence could improve everything from grief counseling to hospice care.

Some of that work has already begun. Over the past decade, people across the country have started congregating in Death Cafés, informal get-togethers over coffee and cake with the purpose of talking about death. Even before the COVID-19 pandemic, more and more people were filling out advance care directives and having discussions with loved ones about their end-of-life wishes. Enabled in part by the nationwide expansion of hospice services, there is a renewed focus on trying to die at home surrounded by loved ones rather than in a hospital.

The desire to die well is part of a growing social movement to wrest back control over life's final chapter from the domain of the medical and funeral profession.[3] Refusing to be stifled by convention, millennials and

THE DAY I DIE

baby boomers are the generations spearheading these efforts.[4] They are the ones researching their options for green burial, natural home death care, aqua-cremation, composting human remains, and turning ashes into tree soil. They write their own eulogies and obituaries, hold living wakes to say goodbye, craft playlists for their funerals, and design their own coffins. Some have found inspiration in the burgeoning "death-positive" movement, which attempts to normalize discussions around our mortality.[5]

But we will also want to be careful not to turn having a "good death" into yet another obligation of late-modern life—a productive life followed by a successful death. Nor should dying well become a luxury reserved for the chosen few with the resources to make it happen. So often, our quick-fix culture demands ready-made solutions for all manner of human suffering. We must ensure that assisted dying continues to be driven by the needs of seriously ill patients and that it remains just one of many ways to have a humane, dignified death.

We might reflect on Barbara Ehrenreich's point that not everything in life can be subject to our mastery. "No matter how much effort we expend," she writes in *Natural Causes*, "not everything is potentially within our control, not even our own bodies and minds."[6]

Bruce learned that lesson the hardest possible way. On August 11, 2020, an email from him popped up in my inbox.

"Hi, hope things are going well with you. Update on out here. I have been diagnosed with pancreatic cancer. Of course, I'm electing no treatment. 1 1/2 years life expectancy. I have sponsors for new bills in 2021. Hope we do better. How is the writing coming along? Thank you for everything, Bruce."

During a routine MRI scan two weeks prior, physicians had detected an aggressive form of pancreatic cancer. The tumor was wrapped around an artery to the liver, which meant that surgery would be too risky. The oncologist told Bruce that he had a 15 percent chance of the tumor decreasing with chemotherapy but that it would inevitably return. Bruce and Kathy pored over survival statistics for pancreatic cancer, realizing quickly that the outlook was grim—even with treatment. They found out that the five-year survival rate for someone in his state was less than 6 percent. Bruce didn't like those odds, so he declined treatment.

Initially, his gastroenterologist had given him a prognosis of a year and a half. When he saw the oncologist two weeks later, his projected timeline shrank down to six months. The news came as a shock to Bruce and Kathy. But it also cleared his path toward an assisted death. In an ironic twist of fate, Bruce could now take advantage of Oregon's Death with Dignity law after years of trying to gain access. He had hit the magical six-month number.

Bruce immediately applied for the law and opted to receive the medication right away. At the end of August, during his hospice intake, his timeline contracted once more. His nurse told him that, based on her experience with pancreatic cancer patients, he could expect to die within three to four months. Because the pancreas is not enveloped by a membrane like the rest of the gastrointestinal organs, pancreatic cancer tends to spread quickly. If there was anything he still wanted to do, now was the time.

The very next week, Bruce took off on a road trip to his hometown in California to bid his old friends goodbye. When he returned weeks later, his nurse increased his daily medication regimen, and Bruce had to give up driving. He set December 1 as the date for his death.

On October 18, Bruce gave a final talk at his local Unitarian church, a cornerstone of his activism the previous few years.

"It's pathetic that I had to get a diagnosis of pancreatic cancer so that I would have a peaceful ending of life," Bruce proclaimed as he clasped the podium. He wore a striped, marine-blue polo shirt, which blended in with the ocean canvas behind him. "But I'm the lucky one. I am lucky. How many of you have always wanted to die in your sleep? I get to *do* that. I get to watch my loved one or *M*A*S*H* or whatever the heck I want as I close my eyes and die."

Bruce told his audience that the three bills that had failed to amend Oregon's Death with Dignity Act in 2019 would be reintroduced in 2021. He finished with an urgent plea.

"If you want to protect yourselves and your future and have a nice, peaceful ending of life where *you* control it, talk to your legislators. It can be done. And this is the year it *should* be done."

Around the time of his final public appearance, Bruce went on liquid morphine. That was when the hallucinations started. Kathy remembered sitting on the bed with him one day as he exploded into uncontrollable giggles. He told Kathy that he had watched Ozzy, one of their small dogs, fetch a pancake for her. Bruce made his wife promise that she wouldn't tell the hospice nurses about his delusions. He didn't want to jeopardize his ability to take the lethal medication.

At the beginning of November, one month before he planned to die, Bruce suddenly had a change of heart. Out of the blue, he told Kathy that he would not use the fatal drugs. After years of fighting for the right to end his life, he decided against it. He planned to die peacefully in his sleep.

"Nobody was more surprised than I was," Kathy recalled.

Bruce never told her why he had changed his mind. But Kathy had a theory.

"It's easy to say what you think you would do when you're not faced with the actual decision to end your own life," Kathy told me. "Bruce was very angry with his diagnosis. He felt he had business he wanted to complete, in terms of Death with Dignity, and I think he felt angry that his life was being cut short. He felt cheated and not—not ready. Bruce loved life. He really did. He didn't want to go."

A few weeks later, at around the time when he had wanted to die, Bruce lost his cognitive functions. As the cancer took over and his drug regimen intensified, he grew unable to make decisions. The drugs that were supposed to calm him down had the opposite effect. He became agitated and restless, and he would be awake almost all night. He developed severe dyskinesia—erratic, involuntary body movements—and his feet became painfully swollen from fluid buildup. Increasingly sensitive to noise, he no longer allowed his beloved dogs into the bedroom. If Bruce had had a crystal ball and could have seen the path he was headed down, said Kathy, he would have taken the lethal medication.

The tipping point came when Bruce's liver started failing in early December. His skin turned jaundiced. His caloric intake plummeted. From then on, Kathy felt that she was always one step behind where she needed to be. One Friday, she called hospice to request a shower assist. By Monday, she canceled the request—she could no longer get Bruce into the shower. Instead, she asked for a wheelchair to be delivered to the house. By the time it arrived, Bruce was already bedbound, so Kathy had to call again and request a lift assist.

Because of Parkinson's, Bruce couldn't use the standard hospice drugs to alleviate his pain and anxiety. Ativan increased his delusions and made him unsteady on his feet; he had several serious falls after taking the medication. One of his hospice nurses recommended that Kathy use Haldol, a drug normally contraindicated for Parkinson's patients. Desperate to find some relief for her husband, Kathy gave it a try.

Bruce's body reacted worse than she could have imagined. His face contorted into a frozen, wide-eyed grimace—it reminded her of *The Scream*, the Edvard Munch painting.

"His muscles completely locked up on him. It was one of the most horrible things I've ever seen. I'm still angry about it."

Around Christmas, Kathy was administering pain medications to Bruce every hour. With secretions and mucus building up in his lungs, Bruce would bolt awake from his slumber and erupt into a violent hacking fit that sent him into a wild panic. Kathy said it sounded like he was trying to cough up a bathtub. At long last, hospice found the right mix of medications to put him into a deep sleep. On Christmas Eve, around seven in the evening, Bruce took his last breath.

"It was not the death that he fought for or envisioned for himself," said Kathy, exhausted from having relived the trauma of Bruce's final weeks.

Yet there was one thought that gave her comfort and allowed her to reframe Bruce's death for herself.

"If I think about the big picture, his fight was all about having a choice. And he did."

EPILOGUE

When I began this project, my personal experience with death was limited. I vaguely recalled the death of two great-grandmothers, a classmate in primary school who died from leukemia, and a cousin who was killed in a train accident. Every once in a while, I received fleeting reminders of my mortality during adventures in the outdoors, but I never had any truly close calls. Like most people, I didn't devote much time to contemplating death. I was too busy sopping up life.

As I stepped into this research, all that changed. Suddenly, I couldn't stop thinking about death. For the first time ever, I wondered what it would feel like to die. The more time I spent with people who were facing the end of their life, the more I questioned our cultural silence around death—and its corrosive effects. We can spend our entire lives studying everything from mathematics to home repair, yet we don't bother learning about one of the most significant events we will ever experience. Speaking with people about how they prepared for death, what they thought about it, and how they grieved didn't feel dark. Uncorking the bottle of our collective death denial felt like an act of liberation.

When I sat down to write this book, death was everywhere. As the coronavirus marched through the country, we kept a public tally of those who had lost their lives. Many of us turned into amateur scientists to compute what level of risk we were willing to tolerate and where we would draw the line. Almost overnight, the specter of mortality began haunting how our bodies moved through space—the way we stepped into the street to avoid a breath that still lingered, dodged doorknobs contaminated by the touch of others, instinctively recoiled at the sound of a cough. And yet our newfound awareness of death didn't seem to make us any less afraid of dying—if anything, it made us more fearful.

In the summer of 2020, death hit closer to home for me. That was when my grandmother plunged from the fourth story of her Soviet-style high rise. Around five o'clock in the morning, she rose from her sleep, put on her sweatpants, slipped through the door to the balcony, placed her house shoes under a chair, climbed onto the seat, and stepped over the railing. A neighbor found her two hours later and notified her husband, still asleep in their bed. He rushed downstairs to find his fatally injured wife next to a shrub. There was no note, no warning, and no explanation. My grandmother suffered from an array of health issues, but she never talked about any of them—she thought it unseemly. At eighty-one years old, my grandmother still dyed her hair a rich chestnut brown to adhere to a culturally sanctioned narrative of agelessness. She took her pain to the grave with her, leaving behind a world of hurt.

A few months later, the week that Oregon was choked by massive wildfires, I lost the child that had been growing inside me for fourteen weeks. As I stared at the frozen bean on the ultrasound screen, three clinicians came and went without telling me the truth of what they saw. A fourth one finally broached the news, through two layers of masks. I don't know how I would have coped with the depth of my grief without having spent all this time studying death—or without being able to bring my pain into the open. Intuitively, I grasped for the power of ritual to mark this sudden and incomprehensible ending. I held a backyard ceremony with close friends to honor the lost soul, and Derianna came and read a poem. We lit candles and floated them in a bowl of water, and one of my friends led us in song. My neighbor built a small wooden display box for the knitted booties I had picked out. I had never felt so held in my life.

The people at the center of this book radically deepened my willingness and capacity to engage with death. They taught me what we, as a culture, stand to gain when we overcome fear and denial and marinate in the truth of our shared mortality. At this point in my life, being silent about death no longer seems like an appealing option.

This book is a snapshot of a moment in time. Since I began writing it, some of the formulas for the life-ending drugs have changed, and some laws are undergoing minor revisions. But the basic contours of what it's like to have an assisted death in America are the same. Formidable barriers to access remain. The letter of the law continues to stifle patients who are either too sick or not sick enough to qualify for a prescription. And physicians who have committed their careers to helping relieve suffering at the end of life face suspicion and critique.

As a society, we can and should do better. As we continue to grapple with the fallout from a global pandemic, we have reached a critical turning point where the contemplation of our mortality becomes ever more closely personal. At this threshold, we have the opportunity to do things differently and chart a more compassionate way forward.

Because ultimately, this all ends. And when it does, having options for what that might look like seems like a kind way to go.

Acknowledgments

It feels overwhelming to think of all the people who have helped bring this book into the world. I owe my deepest thanks to the patients, families, volunteers, physicians, and activists who gave me their time and trusted me with their stories. Though I could include only a small fraction of their voices, our conversations indelibly shaped my understanding of all the stakes and hard labor involved in an assisted death.

A big thanks to Cindy Rasmussen for paving my first foray into the world of assisted dying and becoming such a close friend since then. The volunteers and doctors from End of Life Choices Oregon and End of Life Washington were unwavering supporters of this project from day one, and I thank them sincerely for allowing me access into their world.

Derianna Mooney remains a true force of nature, and I feel so grateful for her friendship and tutelage over the years. Jill and Tony Daniels contributed to this work in more ways than I could ever count—without them, this book wouldn't exist. Among my fellow "deathlings," I want to thank Heather Massey especially, who took me by the hand and introduced me to the wondrous world of natural death care and Death Cafés.

I am indebted to Kemlo Aki and Jenny Nash at Author Accelerator who helped me transform my academic impulses into literary ones and find my own voice. My talented agent, Mackenzie Brady Watson, and her extraordinary team at Stuart Krichevsky Literary Agency showed infinite enthusiasm for this project from the start and have expertly steered it forward since. I thank Anna Michels, my brilliant editor at Sourcebooks, for taking a chance on this book and for always having the right instincts. I am so grateful to her and her team, especially Bridget McCarthy and Liz Kelsch, for being such fierce advocates of this work.

I thank my research assistants who helped me transcribe and weed through my materials over the years: Ilana Cohen, Douglas Bafford, Amanda Votta, Sierra Dakin Kuiper, and Jess Priestley. For the writing and research of this book, I received generous funding from Brandeis University, including from the Provost Research Grant, the Mandel Faculty Grant in the Humanities, and the Theodore and Jane Norman Fund for Faculty Research and Creative Projects. Special thanks to my wonderful colleagues and students at Brandeis who taught me—and continue to teach me—how to integrate academic rigor with creativity and boldness.

I feel intensely grateful to my friends and family, who let me talk about death for years and carried me through all the highs and lows of this project. I owe them everything. Among them, Abram Rosenthal became my indispensable part-time muse, and Jade Giotta, my intrepid, beautiful soul sister, always lit the way. Thank you, all, from the depths of my heart.

Reading Group Guide

1. What had you heard about assisted dying before reading *The Day I Die?* What were you most interested to learn about it? What did you find most surprising?

2. In taking an anthropological approach, Hannig becomes an active participant in several assisted deaths as part of her research. What does this immersive methodology add to the book?

3. Of the people profiled in the book, whom did you find most relatable? What part of their story resonated with you?

4. The story of Joe (the ALS patient from chapters 1 and 9) showcases many of the complications involved in pursuing an assisted death with a neurodegenerative diagnosis. Which obstacle stood out most to you? What do you think could be done to reduce the

hardships faced by people like Joe who would like to die on their own terms?

5. The ability to ingest the life-ending medication yourself is a critical moral and legal pillar of assisted dying laws in America. How do you interpret this requirement? Do you think it is worthwhile to keep it, even if it prevents some patients from using the law?

6. One of the most common arguments against assisted dying is the "slippery slope" that could result from expanded access (discussed in chapter 3). Do you think there's validity to that argument? How does current legislation attempt to prevent such a scenario?

7. Activist John Kelly asserts that medical assistance in dying implicitly devalues the lives of people with disabilities, who must live daily with the same sorts of limitations terminally ill patients try to escape by seeking an assisted death. How can we better support Americans with disabilities? How would you address some of their concerns about assisted dying?

8. Patients who pursue assisted dying often confront a pervasive cultural silence around death, both inside the medical profession but also more broadly. What have you observed about this tendency to deny death in America? Are you familiar with different approaches toward human mortality, perhaps from other cultural contexts?

9. The American Medical Association claims that assisted dying "is fundamentally incompatible with the physician's role as healer." How do the physicians profiled in this book reconcile their involvement in assisted deaths with their role as healers?

10. Families frequently serve as a vital source of support for someone's quest for an assisted death. At the same time, the end of life can further exacerbate long-simmering family tensions. What struck you about some of the family dynamics in this book?

11. One positive effect of an assisted death is its potential for simplifying grief for a decedent's loved ones. What do you think is the most complicated part of grief? How does an assisted death affect that aspect of grieving?

12. *The Day I Die* introduces a variety of personal philosophies around death and dying. Which of these philosophies spoke to you the most? Have they changed how you think about life's final chapter?

13. Many organizations that advocate for assisted dying laws are currently opposed to amendments so as not to endanger the legalization process in other states. Do you think states should continue to wait to update their legislation until assisted dying is more widely accessible or revise their laws now to make them less onerous to use? What are the pros and cons of each approach?

14. After reading, do you think you would ever pursue an assisted death if faced with a terminal diagnosis? What would a "good death" look like to you?

A Conversation with the Author

How did you first become involved with assisted dying? Were you, like Derianna, trying to reframe your own relationship with death?

I actually fell into this subject by accident. I was showing *How to Die in Oregon* (the best documentary on assisted dying, I think) in one of my anthropology classes at Brandeis, and I became immediately hooked. My previous research had been on birth and the beginning of life in Ethiopia, and it felt fitting to change focus and look at the opposite of that. Of course, I soon realized that death was not the opposite of birth but very much akin to it.

How did you build your network of interview subjects?

Initially, I attended public hearings on assisted dying and would approach people afterward to ask for a personal interview. After my first few interviews, people would refer me to other key figures in the movement and pass me around. Once I moved to Oregon, I had interviews scheduled almost every day. Eventually, some of the physicians I met offered to put me in touch with their patients, most of whom were really eager to share their stories. I was astonished by this deep desire to be heard, especially during such a sensitive time.

It's growing more common for people to prepare advance directives and communicate their end-of-life wishes to their families. Do you have any recommendations for beginning those conversations?

Definitely. There is a wealth of resources out there on how to start those conversations. My favorite sites are Death over Dinner (deathoverdinner.org), the Conversation Project (theconversationproject.org), and end-of-life planning tools like Lantern (www.lantern.co).

You've talked to many activists who are both for and against access to assisted dying. Do you think we're likely to see assisted dying legislation in all fifty states any time soon?

Not any time soon, unless the U.S. Supreme Court reverses its 1997 ruling that the right to die is *not* protected by the Constitution (leaving it up to individual states to design their own laws). If we had a federal recognition of the right to die, similar to the federal recognition of same-sex marriage in 2015, then I think we could see assisted dying legislation in all fifty states.

You discuss your anthropological approach to writing this book as a matter of immersion. What does that level of immersion add to your research? What makes immersion most difficult?

I think that all human experience is inherently subjective and that we can't ever fully think ourselves into someone else's shoes. The closest we can get is undergoing a small part of that experience with someone else—not as a passive bystander but as an active participant. Experiencing an assisted death alongside a patient and their family gives you a much deeper level of insight than hearing about it secondhand. It's a very visceral and transformative experience. I sometimes struggled with feeling like an intruder during such tender moments, until I realized that folks welcomed my presence. They appreciated that I showed up wholeheartedly and became a part of everything that happened rather than standing on the sidelines.

You mention some of the ways the COVID-19 pandemic has changed people's approach to death. Did it affect the way you wrote *The Day I Die?* If so, how?

The pandemic made me even more aware of how difficult it is for many people to contend with the topic of death. I thought a lot about how to break through to readers who have been avoiding the subject so far. In the end, I decided that the best way to talk about death was through the eyes of my protagonists and how they grappled with their own mortality. It felt important to show that death isn't always unambiguously tragic but can also be full of beauty and grace.

What does your writing process look like? Do you have any writing rituals?

I have lots of writing rituals (some might call them neuroses). I sit down to write first thing in the morning with a cup of green tea and listen to the same quiet classical music while I settle into the work. Once I have something on the page, I comb through every sentence and try to make it more concise, cutting any excess weight. Then I do the same at the paragraph level. I spend as much—if not more—time revising as I do writing. If I get stuck, I take myself outside for some fresh air. Usually, the right phrase will come to me then.

What books are on your bedside table these days?

I am fascinated by the potential of psychedelics to relieve fear of death at the end of life, especially for terminally ill patients. So I am reading Michael Pollan's *How to Change Your Mind*. Besides that, I find levity and thrill in books on local backpacking adventures.

Resources

For general information on assisted dying laws and initiatives in your state:

https://www.compassionandchoices.org/
https://deathwithdignity.org/

For practical information on the assisted dying pathway for patients and clinicians:

https://www.acamaid.org/

For volunteer organizations that assist patients and caregivers in select states:

California: https://endoflifechoicesca.org/
Maine: https://www.mainedeathwithdignity.org/

New Mexico: https://endoflifeoptionsnm.org/

Oregon: https://eolcoregon.org/

Vermont: https://www.patientchoices.org/

Washington: https://endoflifewa.org/

For more information on hospice and palliative care services nationwide:

https://www.nhpco.org/

Notes

Introduction: A New Way to Die

1   "Death with Dignity Legislation," Frequently Asked Questions, Death with Dignity, accessed July 20, 2021, https://deathwithdignity.org/faqs/#laws.

2   Megan Brenan, "Americans' Strong Support for Euthanasia Persists," Gallup, May 31, 2018, https://news.gallup.com/poll/235145/americans-strong-support-euthanasia-persists.aspx.

3   "Euthanasia Bill Moves Ahead in Spanish Parliament," Reuters, February 11, 2020, https://www.reuters.com/article/us-spain-politics-euthanasia/euthanasia-bill-moves-ahead-in-spanish-parliament-idUSKBN2052C0.

4   "Deaths by Manner of Death and County of Residence, Oregon Residents 2018 Final Data," Oregon Health Authority, https://www.oregon.gov/oha/PH/BIRTHDEATHCERTIFICATES/VITALSTATISTICS/DEATH/Documents/dman18.pdf; Public Health Division, Center for Health Statistics, "Oregon Death with Dignity Act: 2018 Data Summary," Oregon Health Authority, revised April 25, 2019, https://www.oregon.gov/oha/PH/PROVIDERPARTNERRESOURCES/EVALUATIONRESEARCH/DEATHWITHDIGNITYACT/Documents/year21.pdf.

5   In the last seven years, five feature films have come out on assisted dying—*The Farewell Party* (2014), *Me Before You* (2016), *Paddleton* (2019), *Blackbird* (2019),

Here Awhile (2020)—and major TV series like *Grey's Anatomy* and *Grace and Frankie* dedicated entire episodes to it.

6   Atul Gawande, *Being Mortal: Medicine and What Matters in the End* (New York: Penguin, 2014), 58.

7   In practice, physicians in Montana follow the letter of the Oregon law because they don't have their own.

8   Public Health Division, Center for Health Statistics, "Oregon Death with Dignity Act: 2020 Data Summary," Oregon Health Authority, February 26, 2021, https://www.oregon.gov/oha/PH/PROVIDERPARTNERRESOURCES /EVALUATIONRESEARCH/DEATHWITHDIGNITYACT/Documents /year23.pdf.

9   "Oregon Death with Dignity Act: 2020 Data Summary."

10   Census QuickFacts for Oregon from July 1, 2019, United States Census Bureau, https://www.census.gov/quickfacts/fact/table/OR/PST045219.

11   Census QuickFacts for California from July 1, 2019, United States Census Bureau, https://www.census.gov/quickfacts/CA; "California End of Life Option Act 2019 Data Report," California Department of Public Health, July 2022, https://www.cdph.ca.gov/Programs/CHSI/CDPH%20Document%20Library /CDPHEndofLifeOptionActReport2019%20_Final%20ADA.pdf.

12   Amber E. Barnato et al., "Racial and Ethnic Differences in Preferences for End-of-Life Treatment," *Journal of General Internal Medicine* 24, no. 6 (2009): 695–701, https://doi.org/10.1007/s11606-009-0952-6.

13   The historical record is saturated with instances of medical maltreatment of and experimentation on people of color. For a short selection: Harriet A. Washington, *Medical Apartheid: The Dark History of Medical Experimentation on Black Americans from Colonial Times to the Present* (New York: Doubleday, 2007) and Deirdre Cooper Owens, *Medical Bondage: Race, Gender, and the Origins of American Gynecology* (Athens: University of Georgia Press, 2017).

14   Nathan A. Boucher et al., "Palliative Care in the African American Community," Palliative Care Network of Wisconsin, 2019, https://www.mypcnow.org/fast-fact /palliative-care-in-the-african-american-community/. See also: Kimberly S. Johnson, "Racial and Ethnic Disparities in Palliative Care," *Journal of Palliative Medicine* 16, no. 11 (2013): 1329–34, https://doi.org/10.1089/jpm.2013.9468.

15   "Health Disparities by Race and Ethnicity: The California Landscape," California

Health Care Almanac, October 2019, https://www.chcf.org/wp-content /uploads/2019/10/DisparitiesAlmanacRaceEthnicity2019.pdf.

16   "Religious Landscape Study: Racial and Ethnic Composition," Pew Research Center (2014), https://www.pewforum.org/religious-landscape-study/racial-and-ethnic -composition/; Kimberly S. Johnson, Katja Elbert-Avila, and James A. Tulsky, "The Influence of Spiritual Beliefs and Practices on the Treatment Preferences of African Americans: A Review of the Literature," *Journal of the American Geriatrics Society* 53, no. 4 (2005): 711–19, https://doi.org/10.1111/j.1532-5415.2005.53224.x.

17   Shirley A. Hill, "Ethnicity and the Ethic of Caring in African American Families," *Journal of Personal and Interpersonal Loss* 2, no. 2 (1996): 109–28, https://doi .org/10.1080/10811449708414410; Anne Streaty Wimberly, *Honoring African American Elders: A Ministry in the Soul Community* (San Francisco: Jossey-Bass, 1997); Jung Kwak and William E. Haley, "Current Research Findings on End-of-Life Decision Making among Racially or Ethnically Diverse Groups," *Gerontologist* 45, no. 5 (2005): 634–41, https://doi.org/10.1093/geront/45.5.634.

18   Private insurance companies differ on whether they fund the cost of life-ending medication and physician appointments. Oregon's Medicaid insurance, the Oregon Health Plan, does cover life-ending medication, but patients typically have to pay up front and hope their family will be reimbursed later on. Federally funded insurance programs, such as Medicare or Veterans Affairs, don't pay for the medication because federal monies may not be used to cover expenses related to assisted dying. As the majority of patients who use Oregon's law are over the age of sixty-five, their default insurance tends to be Medicare, which means they must cover the cost of the medication themselves. If patients can get their prescriber to bill their insurance for a general end-of-life consultation (even under Medicare) or if doctors volunteer their time, then patients can defray the cost of their medical appointments, which may run up to $5,000.

Chapter 1: Spinning Away

1   Susan Sontag, *Illness as Metaphor and AIDS and Its Metaphors* (New York: Picador, 2001), 99.

Chapter 2: When Hospice Isn't Enough

1   "Where Do Americans Die?" Palliative Care, Stanford School of Medicine, https://palliative.stanford.edu/home-hospice-home-care-of-the-dying-patient/where-do-americans-die/.

2   Katy Butler, *The Art of Dying Well: A Practical Guide to a Good End of Life* (New York: Scribner, 2019), 8.

3   The American Academy of Hospice and Palliative Medicine has adopted a position of "studied neutrality" toward assisted dying. For their full statement: http://aahpm.org/positions/pad.

4   David Marchese, "COVID Has Traumatized America. A Doctor Explains What We Need to Heal," *New York Times*, March 24, 2021, https://www.nytimes.com/interactive/2021/03/22/magazine/diane-e-meier-interview.html.

5   Jim Parker, "Lack of Palliative Care Definition Impacts Patients, Hospice Business," Hospice News, November 1, 2019, https://hospicenews.com/2019/11/01/lack-of-palliative-care-definition-impacts-patients-hospice-business/.

6   Thanks to Michael Pottash for this apt characterization.

7   Aleccia JoNel, "Where You Live May Determine How You Die, Study Suggests," Kaiser Health News, March 15, 2017, https://www.statnews.com/2017/03/15/death-end-of-life-states/.

8   "Oregon Death with Dignity Act: 2020 Data Summary."

9   As sociologist Shai Lavi notes, "What makes the practice of [palliative sedation] unique is that it was institutionalized without undergoing any legal, moral, or public scrutiny." Shai J. Lavi, *The Modern Art of Dying: A History of Euthanasia in the United States* (Princeton, NJ: Princeton University Press, 2005), 127.

10 In 1994, the Supreme Court case *Vacco v. Quill* upheld the double effect doctrine in support of aggressive pain management and palliative sedation at the end of life.

Chapter 3: Restrictive Laws

1   The interview was conducted by Matthew E. Simek as part of a project by the Oregon Health and Science University Oral History Program on June 4, 2008. In 2012, Goodwin used the Death with Dignity Act himself after being diagnosed with a rare neurodegenerative disease.

2   For the full letter of the Oregon Death with Dignity Act: https://www.oregon.gov

/oha/ph/providerpartnerresources/evaluationresearch/deathwithdignityact
/Pages/ors.aspx.

3   In Hawaii, these include requiring a mandatory mental health exam and a twenty-day waiting period in between oral requests.

4   While recently passed assisted dying legislation in Victoria, Western Australia, and New Zealand comes close to the U.S. model, these laws are still more permissive than U.S. laws. They allow a medical practitioner to administer the lethal medication if a patient is unable or unwilling to self-administer the drugs. Laws in Victoria and Western Australia also permit a twelve-month terminal prognosis for neurodegenerative diseases.

5   Richard N. Côté, *In Search of Gentle Death: The Fight for Your Right to Die with Dignity* (Mt. Pleasant, SC: Corinthian Books, 2012), 243.

6   "Fourth Interim Report on Medical Assistance in Dying in Canada," Health Canada, April 2019, https://www.canada.ca/en/health-canada/services/publications /health-system-services/medical-assistance-dying-interim-report-april-2019.html.

7   Ari Gandsman, "'A Recipe for Elder Abuse:' From Sin to Risk in Anti-Euthanasia Activism," *Death Studies* 40, no. 9 (October 2016): 578–88, https://doi.org/10.108 0/07481187.2016.1193568.

8   Oregon's Death with Dignity Act does not require a medical provider to be present at an assisted death. However, it does require that the attending physician counsel the patient on the importance of having another person present when they take the lethal medication.

9   Faced with a lack of legal guidance, some doctors' offices and volunteer organizations have designed their own directives that patients fill out prior to an assisted death. The forms explain that there is a small risk that the medication won't have the intended effect. A patient can check one of two options: regain consciousness with the understanding that their mental or physical functioning may not return to previous levels or receive additional sedatives to keep them unconscious until they die.

Chapter 4: Invisible Death

1   Caitlin Doughty, *Smoke Gets in Your Eyes: And Other Lessons from the Crematory* (New York: W. W. Norton, 2014), 234.

2   Gawande, *Being Mortal*, 8–9.

3   Philippe Ariès, "The Hour of Our Death," in *Death, Mourning, and Burial*, ed. Antonius C. G. M. Robben (New York: Blackwell, 2004), 47.

4   Rupert Stasch, *Society of Others: Kinship and Mourning in a West Papuan Place* (Berkeley: University of California Press, 2009), 208.

5   Caitlin Doughty, *From Here to Eternity: Traveling the World to Find the Good Death* (New York: W. W. Norton, 2017), 77–104.

6   Daniel Callahan, "Reason, Self-Determination, and Physician-Assisted Suicide," in *The Case Against Assisted Suicide: For the Right to End-of-Life Care*, ed. Kathleen Foley and Herbert Hendin (Baltimore: Johns Hopkins University Press, 2002), 52–68; Paul T. Schotsmans, "Relational Responsibility, and Not Only Stewardship: A Roman Catholic View on Voluntary Euthanasia for Dying and Non-Dying Patients," *Christian Bioethics* 9, nos. 2–3 (August–December 2003): 285–98, https://doi.org/10.1076/chbi.9.2.285.30288.

7   Ian Hacking, "The Suicide Weapon," *Critical Inquiry* 35, no. 1 (2008): 1–32, https://doi.org/10.1086/595626.

8   Marilyn Golden and Tyler Zoanni, "Killing Us Softly: The Dangers of Legalizing Assisted Suicide," *Disability and Health Journal* 3, no. 1 (January 2010): 16–30, https://doi.org/10.1016/j.dhjo.2009.08.006.

9   This policy has also prevented life insurance companies from reneging on their policies. Even though the death certificate doesn't mention assisted dying, prescribing physicians in most states must file detailed paperwork for each case with the state.

10   Peter Goodwin, interview by Matthew E. Simek, Oregon Health and Sciences University, Oral History Program, June 4, 2008.

11   John Michael Bostwick and Lewis M. Cohen, "Differentiating Suicide from Life-Ending Acts and End-of-Life Decisions: A Model Based on Chronic Kidney Disease and Dialysis," *Psychosomatics* 50, no.1 (January–February 2009): 1–7, https://doi.org/10.1176/appi.psy.50.1.1.

12   "Oregon Death with Dignity Act: 2020 Data Summary."

13   Lavi, *Modern Art of Dying*, 15.

14   Gawande, *Being Mortal*, 157. Atul Gawande asks, "How do you attend to the thoughts and concerns of the dying when medicine has made it almost impossible to be sure who the dying even are?"

Chapter 6: Medical Gatekeepers

1   "Oregon Death with Dignity Act: 2020 Data Summary"; Frédéric Michas, "Number of Active Physicians in Oregon 2020, by Specialty Area," Statista, June 5, 2020.

2   Gawande, *Being Mortal*, 169.

3   For AMA's full statement: https://www.ama-assn.org/delivering-care/ethics /physician-assisted-suicide.

4   Giza Lopes, *Dying with Dignity: A Legal Approach to Assisted Death* (Santa Barbara: Praeger, 2015), 78–80.

5   Nicholas A. Christakis, *Death Foretold: Prophecy and Prognosis in Medical Care* (Chicago: University of Chicago Press, 1999), xv.

6   Christakis, *Death Foretold*, xii.

7   Paul Glare et al., "A Systematic Review of Physicians' Survival Predictions in Terminally Ill Cancer Patients," *British Medical Journal* 327, no. 7408 (July 2003): 195–98, https://doi.org/10.1136/bmj.327.7408.195.

8   "Oregon Death with Dignity Act: 2020 Data Summary."

9   Besides suffering from a mental disorder, people commit suicide based on a variety of situational reasons (being fired from a job, facing a public scandal, unrequited love), which may cause acute emotional despair.

10   "Oregon Death with Dignity Act: 2020 Data Summary."

Chapter 7: The Science of Dying

1   "Oregon Death with Dignity Act: 2020 Data Summary."

2   "Oregon Death with Dignity Act: 2020 Data Summary."

3   "Oregon Death with Dignity Act: 2020 Data Summary."

4   Robert Desjarlais, *Subject to Death: Life and Loss in a Buddhist World* (Chicago: University of Chicago Press, 2016); Scott Stonington, *The Spirit Ambulance: Choreographing the End of Life in Thailand* (Berkeley: University of California Press, 2020).

Chapter 8: Family Matters

1   Talal Asad, *Formations of the Secular: Christianity, Islam, and Modernity* (Palo Alto: Stanford University Press, 2003), 82.

Chapter 9: Flying Free

1   "Oregon Death with Dignity Act: 2020 Data Summary."

2   Christina Nicolaidis, "My Mother's Choice," *Journal of the American Medical Association* 296, no. 8 (2006): 907–8, https://doi.org/10.1001/jama.296.8.907.

Chapter 10: Crossing Over

1   Desjarlais, *Subject to Death*, 50.

2   Vicky Bach, Jenny Ploeg, and Margaret Black, "Nursing Roles in End-of-Life Decision Making in Critical Care Settings," *Western Journal of Nursing Research* 31, no. 4 (June 2009): 496–512, https://doi.org/10.1177/0193945908331178.

Chapter 11: Together in Grief

1   Deborah Schwing and Leslie Dennett, "Grief Outcomes in Medical Aid in Dying," conference paper presented at the National Clinicians Conference on Medical Aid in Dying, Berkeley, California, February 15, 2020.

2   Linda Ganzini et al., "Mental Health Outcomes of Family Members of Oregonians Who Request Physician Aid in Dying," *Journal of Pain and Symptom Management* 38, no. 6 (December 2009): 807–15, https://doi.org/10.1016/j.jpainsymman.2009.04.026.

3   Desjarlais, *Subject to Death*, 115.

4   Maurice Bloch, "Death, Women, and Power," in *Death and the Regeneration of Life*, ed. Maurice Bloch and Jonathan Parry (Cambridge: Cambridge University Press, 1982), 211–30.

Chapter 12: New Frontiers

1   Oregon HB 2232, Oregon Legislative Assembly–2019 Regular Session, https://legiscan.com/OR/text/HB2232/id/1843939.

2   Mark Mather, Paola Scommegna, and Lillian Kilduff, "Fact Sheet: Aging in the United States," *Population Bulletin* 70, no. 2 (July 15, 2019), https://www.prb.org/aging-unitedstates-fact-sheet/.

3   Christine Colby, "These Women Want You to Have a Better Death," *Bust*, August 4,

2017, https://bust.com/feminism/193265-death-positive-movement.html.

4   Eleanor Cummins, "Why Millennials Are the 'Death Positive' Generation," *Vox*, January 22, 2020, https://www.vox.com/the-highlight/2020/1/15/21059189/death-millennials-funeral-planning-cremation-green-positive; Dan Kadlec, "A Good Death: How Boomers Will Change the World a Final Time," *Time*, August 14, 2013, https://business.time.com/2013/08/14/a-good-death-how-boomers-will-change-the-world-a-final-time/.

5   John Leland, "The Positive Death Movement Comes to Life," *New York Times*, June 22, 2018, https://www.nytimes.com/2018/06/22/nyregion/the-positive-death-movement-comes-to-life.html.

6   Barbara Ehrenreich, *Natural Causes: Life, Death, and the Illusion of Control* (New York: Twelve, 2018), xiii.

About the Author

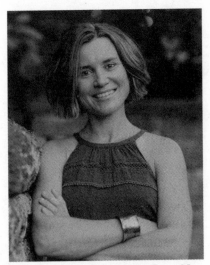

Anita Hannig is associate professor of anthropology at Brandeis University, where she teaches classes on medicine, religion, and death and dying. In recent years, Hannig has emerged as a leading voice on death literacy in America, giving interviews for the *Washington Post*, *USA Today*, and the *Boston Globe*. She is the author of the award-winning book *Beyond Surgery* and has written for *Cognoscenti* and *Undark Magazine*, among others. Her work has been supported by multiple fellowships and grants, including from the Wenner-Gren Foundation and the Mellon Foundation. In her free time, she enjoys trail running, rock climbing, and backpacking in the great outdoors, pursuits that sporadically bring her in touch with her own mortality.